RECLAIM YOUR BRAIN

OPTIMIZE COGNITIVE FUNCTION, PREVENT CHRONIC DISEASE, RESOLVE ANXIETY AND DEPRESSION USING NATURAL METHODS

DR. STRONG D.C. DACNB, CFMP, PAK

"The smartest thing you could ever admit about your health is to acknowledge that your daily run of the mill choices matter; from the food you eat, to the sleep you take, to the love you make – in the long run, you reap tomorrow what you sow today."

— ANON.

CONTENTS

SPECIAL BONUS!

Want These 2 Bonus Books for <u>FREE</u>?

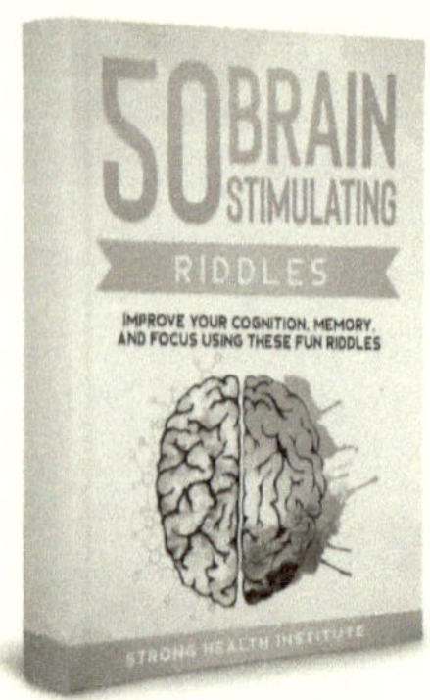

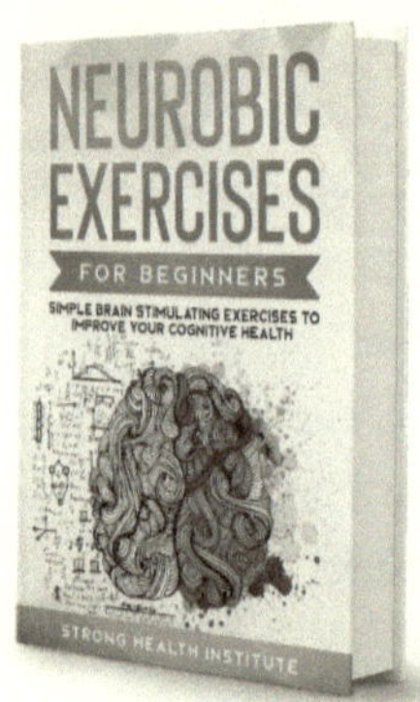

Get <u>FREE</u>, unlimited access to these and all of our new books by joining our community!

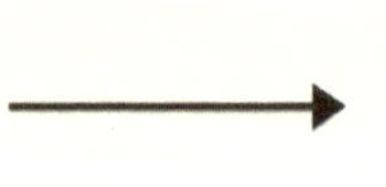

INTRODUCTION

Headaches, migraines, foggy thinking, depression, anxiety, hyper-stress, Alzheimer's, Parkinson's, forgetfulness, losing your mental edge, poor performance at work…

These are the things you might be suffering from right now.

If you, or perhaps someone close to you like a family member, good friend, spouse, or lover are struggling with some of these terrible challenges, then don't give up or lose hope.

I wrote this book just for you!

This book is literally packed with easy to understand and easy to implement tips, tools, and empowering information – to help you to understand what you are going through, learn what contributes to it, and then specifically show you what to do to deal with it directly.

Don't be fooled, "easy" doesn't mean the road ahead will be easy, nor does it mean that this book has dumbed down anything. On the contrary, in the context of modern life, we all need the 'essential' or the 'essence' of something to maximize the potency of our choices, bring about healing changes, and come to balance.

So, if you are struggling with some of the problems I mentioned above, and you are at your wits' end and don't know what to do, then this book can help you by informing you, empowering you, and clearly showing you a way to reclaim your own 'Super Brain'. If the hardest part in healing is learning what you need to do, then this book makes it that much easier – the rest follows on naturally from there.

I wrote this book because after working with many patients in my health practice over the years it struck me that so many of them were suffering from the same or similar troubles. The most heart-wrenching cases always involved serious chronic illnesses like diabetes, heart disease, cancer, and of course the subject of this book, which is gradually degenerating brain health and the associated anxiety and depression that comes with that.

Unbalanced brain functioning and degenerating brain health tended to be one of the most heart-wrenching health challenges for my patients, their friends, and their families to go through. In these sorts of cases, everyone involved, including the patient and their immediate family, have to suffer witnessing the loss of dignity, personality, and pride that comes with a degenerating brain – they literally lose who they are.

Slowly, they transform from who they were into something far less and underserved; moody, angry, depressed, forgetful, drifting ghosts of their former selves. Eventually, the sorrowful truth is that they often die from their conditions. That is one of the most heart-wrenching experiences for a family to go through.

What made it especially tragic for me to witness as a functional medicine doctor was that I knew that these things were largely preventable, manageable, and reversible – significantly so.

I have often found myself thinking in consultation, "If only you had come to me sooner, I could have shared the good news that there are so many things you CAN do to heal, if only you had been given the right information and guidance earlier on".

For me, seeing the families, friends, and loved ones of my patients have to their gradual decline into senescence was, frankly speaking, 'mind-bendingly' heartbreaking.

Nevertheless, not all my patients came to me too late. Many of the people that have come to consult with me about these particular health issues came to me early enough to heal completely. In these cases the advice I gave them was generally the same: they received guidance on how to become healthier, improve their thinking, help ease depression, reduce anxiety, cure migraines, eliminate pain, improve their energy levels, and boost their mental/cognitive performance.

Some even came to me with the early signs of chronic brain illnesses like Alzheimer's, Parkinson's, and the like. But, even then, with the correct information and guidance all of these conditions ended up being manageable in some constructive way - if not completely reversible.

These are the success stories, the ones that fill me with happiness because, at least for a great many people, they managed to recover and spare themselves and their loved ones tremendous amounts of stress, pain, suffering, and anxiety.

The success stories all have a few things in common. They all managed to heal their brains with simple methods that were easy to understand, and easy to do (once understood); and they gradually restored their bodies and minds to balance in a natural healthy way - without the use of potent pharmaceutical drugs, invasive toxic procedures, or expensive biomedical intervention. They just implemented simple empowering daily choices. So you may be wondering what kinds of choices they made.

They made choices like:

- Eating the right foods, avoiding the wrong foods.
- Taking supplements that are smart, efficient, safe, affordable, easily available, and best for your brain. Only taking supplements for as long as necessary, and preferring to transition to a lifestyle of sustainable optimal living in the long run.
- They all made efforts to reduce stress, they began to sleep properly, and insisted on appropriate and wise exercise regimens.
- Systematically healing damaged parts of the body that support the brain – especially optimizing the heart, blood vessels, immune system, and gut.
- Choosing to heal and be healthy for their brain *every single day* - before, during, and after challenging symptoms may have appeared.
- They stayed motivated because they saw the benefits, which led to sticking to their commitment

> to healthy choices, which led to even more benefits
> – transforming the 'downward spiral' of ill health
> into an upward spiral of ever-increasing health and
> wellbeing.

These are the things that really make a difference to your health in general, and to your brain in particular. This is true not only if you are suffering from a medical condition but also if you want to increase your mental performance and become resilient and resistant to illness while healthy, especially as you age.

So, I wrote this book with two aims in mind. The first was to reach a wider audience in the hopes that I would have to see fewer people and their families suffer in my practice. The second was to get the word out there, "You can do something about it, it can get better, and here is how". Getting the word out in this book will definitely help to reach people early and empower them to take charge of their health and create the kind of lives they want as they progress on their paths through life. So, simply speaking, this book is for you.

Why do our brains become dysfunctional? The short and simple answer is that they inevitably start to become dysfunctional because of our day to day choices combined with the stresses and struggles of modern life.

Diet; nutrition; pesticide exposure; modern stress; modern convenience-based sedentary lifestyles of lazy comfort; poor nutritional information; counter-productive medical practices and conflicting profit agendas in health and agriculture – all of these things combine and contribute to us getting ill in the long run. The process happens gradually, insidiously day by day over the span of many years. Eventually, even our astoundingly resilient bodies and brains crumble to the relentless erosive negative health pressures of day-to-day living in modern times - this is the main reason why we become ill with chronic degenerative problems today.

The hard truth is that in a very specific sense you have carefully created the perfect conditions for your illnesses to arise, particularly in the case of long term chronic diseases linked to aging. This happens mostly because people don't know to make better health choices - they may have the wrong information guiding them to mistakenly make poor choices despite doing what they think is correct.

One of the main aims of this book is to correct that horrible mistake, and then to go on to give very clear practical tips and instructions as to the kinds of things you can be doing to support your brain health and mental performance. Gradually, as the years pass by, the little choices you make every day will end up powerfully and radically supporting your health in a positive way.

Throughout our life, we are constantly harnessing the power of our brains and learning how to use them to their full potential. This endlessly complex organ that we call the brain is the control center for everything that makes you tick–from the thoughts in your head down to the movement in your toes. Thus, it would make sense that your brain depends on a nutritional diet, regular exercise, and mindfulness to function at its highest potential.

Your brain did not evolve mechanisms to handle the distractions, empty nutrition, and "mass-produced" stress we're all experiencing in the 21st century. Our bodies evolved their current mechanisms hundreds of thousands of years ago (if not more), they have not really 'caught up' to the pace of modern civilized progress.

Consider that it is commonplace these days to feel the stressful jabs of hundreds of emails, text messages, and "push" notifications, media bombardment, road traffic, pollution, clustered living, and action-packed fully booked schedules, deadlines, and family obligations - all within the context of what has largely become a hyper-competitive modern social context. All of this information is coming at us each day in every single moment we are awake; it overloads us, clouds our focus, and prevents our productivity.

On top of the informational demands on our brain, we often rely heavily on the least nutritionally dense foods. Food that is high in 'convenience', calories, fat, salt, and additives, but low in actual nutrients. These foods are easy to get, fast, and keep us feeling 'full' for longer. But, the illusion of 'fullness' is a dangerous and tempting lie - these foods are really empty and do not support your health, they only push back our hunger temporarily until the next 'hungry moment'.

These foods often contribute to foggy thinking immediately after eating them. I mean, have you ever really considered or questioned why you end up feeling sluggish and drowsy half an hour after eating that take out? These foods feel 'fulfilling', nourishing, nurturing, but the truth is that they are not. Gradually over time, it isn't just the sluggish 'food-comas' 30 minutes after eating that we have to deal with. No, in the long run, these foods actively contribute to nutritional deficiencies, inflammation, obesity, and a host of other problems that directly create conditions in your body that lead to chronic illnesses. If these sluggish impoverished effects are felt by healthy people when they consistently eat these kinds of foods, what do you think the effects would be on people who have underlying health conditions or vulnerabilities? You guessed it, a complete health disaster – especially in the long term.

For people who already have underlying health problems, the situation is compounded and far worse. The adverse effects of eating junk and then dealing with the stresses of daily life toxically combine and magnify all the negative effects on the body. The sad thing is that this happens to the people who can least afford these kinds of consequences – the ones who are already struggling with underlying health problems.

So, it isn't really that surprising that so many of us today open ourselves to a bunch of largely avoidable health issues like failing memory, chronic fatigue, brain fog, depression, anxiety, insomnia, and migraines. When left unchecked, these problems often escalate into serious degenerative diseases; they are actually the early warning signs that your body needs something to change. Without doing things differently, those signs foretell an inevitable health disaster in the form of chronic and debilitating degenerative illness.

So, if you have these signs then it is definitely time to listen to them. In the long run, it is best to acknowledge that your current path leads to a known disastrous health outcome. Once that is acknowledged and really understood, then you will be in a position to look towards changing the end of your story to something more fulfilling and vibrant – radiant health is yours for the taking, just nip the current story in the bud.

Today, more people seem to be struggling with psycholog-ical issues than ever before. Years ago, I too struggled to keep my brain and body fit. As a young adult, I struggled to make the most of my life because I spent so much time fighting against the habitual negative thought patterns my brain seemed to constantly run on loops. Aside from eating poorly, I didn't understand how my brain worked, nor did I know how to take care of it in the way that I needed to. After years of the same daily struggle, I decided I'd finally had enough. Desperate for a solution and motivated to end my suffering, I voraciously researched ways to better myself and I ended up enrolling in medical training to learn about the factors that really affect health.

Years later, now as a professional healer, I've had the good fortune to help literally hundreds of people turn their own lives around and create the health they were all desperately looking for; just as I did.

Through the years, as a functional medicine practitioner, and chiropractic neurologist, I've watched people transform for the better right before my very eyes - I would like to pass on what I've learned to you, this book is my attempt to do that in terms of your brain health – I'd like to help you reclaim your life, your 'self', and "reclaim your brain"!

Throughout this book, I will help you to personally identify the health issues that might be holding you back from having a robust and healthy brain and body. Once identified, you can work with the easy tips and suggestions and concrete plans of action in this book to remove those issues – simple, easy, effective and, of course, healthy.

If left unchecked, memory issues, anxiety, depression, and brain fog can definitely lead to Alzheimer's disease, Parkinson's disease, multiple sclerosis, and other diseases. So, if you begin your journey right now, you can minimize your chances of developing these issues and maximize your opportunities to have a vibrant and fulfilling life.

Even if you have already come to a place in your life where a serious chronic disease has manifested for you, even then, it is never too late to start your healing. Sure, healing from that point is a little more challenging than starting early. But, the truth is I've helped people from all ages and walks of life empower themselves to make incredible progress — even those who previously thought it was too late for them to make a change. Consider one of my patients, Leanne, who thought she had no hope of living pain-free and was at her wit's end; when she came to me she had given up hope, she was literally at her lowest point.

When Leanne first arrived in my practice she was a mother in her late 30s who felt as though her remaining years were numbered. At only 38 years old she had already been diagnosed with fibromyalgia and multiple sclerosis. She was, even then, experiencing daily migraines, chronic pain, high blood pressure, and excessive uncontrollable weight gain. As we ran through the checklist of initial symptoms, she broke down.

How could Leanne be in such a terrible state of health when only a few years before coming to see me she was relatively healthy, lived an active lifestyle, and ran several marathons a year? What happened to her, and why was she in so much daily pain now after only a few short years? The issue was that she missed the early warning signs that her body was giving her, and she had no clue as to what to do – she was just doing the best she knew how.

To help improve her quality of life, Leanne and I worked together to build a diet that supported all her critical body systems that were out of balance and supporting her symptoms. We redesigned her internal states like her gut environment, heart and blood vessels, and her brain by simply helping her to make positive powerful daily choices as well as cleansing the diet of toxic foods, going on a simple nutritional supplement plan, and making sure that her exercise, sleep, stress, and moods were all in good order.

In just one month, she saw results - results that had so far been eluding her. She lost weight, regained hope, and found the energy to start taking daily walks. Slowly, step by step she began to reclaim her body, and brain. Now, she says she has, "never felt better".

Leanne's case was rather extreme, granted, extreme in the sense that her symptoms were severe and extreme in the sense that her recovery was spectacular. But, don't let that make you think that her case doesn't apply to you. On the contrary, it just shows how important the simple daily things are to your overall health and wellness.

The power of changing your diet, supplementation, handling stress, sleeping properly, and exercising appropriately is not to be dismissed casually. For Leanne, those were the only things that actually made any difference.

In the short term, her results kept her motivated. In the long term, she completely healed. Now, she is enjoying her life without the handicap of illness making it harder than it should be – life is hard enough without being ill in the first place.

Leanne's case is extreme, but it isn't far from typical or uncommon. Her story might mirror yours, or contain elements that you are dealing with too. Her story shows that it is never too late (or too severe) to make a massive beneficial difference. You can read more about Leanne's healing journey a little below – I have included it here because her story is one of hope, determination, and success. Her success arose out of the very same methods and information contained in this book.

These methods can help everyone, from healthy people to the most severely ill because they support the critical factors of great brain health. This means that the methods and information in this book actually support the critical factors that can provide empowering opportunities for a life of vibrant energy, radiant health, and long term quality and fulfillment.

This book presents the best good professional advice and tips tailored to your brain health - advice and knowledge gained through my own healing and my years of clinical practical experience. However, in the end, this book will only have any real value to you if you put the information and suggestions into practice in your own life. Only you have the power to reclaim your brain, and although this book will show you how to do that, you need to take the necessary steps. In fact, you have already taken a great first step by picking up this book - It's up to you to take it further, take the next step, one of many, and actively create a better quality of life for yourself – you CAN do it, it starts here. Just as hundreds of my patients have done before, just as Leanne managed to do it for herself, so it is for you too.

LEANNE'S STORY

As mentioned above, Leanne came to me in a bind. In her late 30s, she had been diagnosed with a whole bunch of health issues on top of her experiencing chronic pain, crippling and severe anxiety, and chronic fatigue that destroyed her ability to cope with the demands of day to day life. With her permission, I have included the retelling of her night-and-day transformation from her first-person perspective, which has been edited for length and clarity.

"I remember walking into The Strong Health Institute one day in August of 2019. I wore one of the few outfits I could still fit into—stretchy pants, a t-shirt, and no makeup. I had no confidence that anything said or done by this doctor would be able to help me. I had reached a low in life that I had never experienced before. I was extremely depressed, in chronic pain, and completely without hope."

As we began chatting, I began crying. I wanted to be more present for my children, and I wanted to reclaim my level of health I had in my early 30s when I regularly ran races as long as half marathons. Tearfully, I recounted my medical journey over the years.

"I wasn't sleeping well, I had daily migraines that worsened with time. My hands, feet, and face were so swollen that I was embarrassed to be seen in public. My blood pressure was getting higher every time I checked it. I couldn't concentrate, I had no energy, and I had gained 30 pounds in just one and a half years. An MRI in 2017 showed that I had lesions in my brain, and I was put on two prescription medications for migraines at that time. When I was 36, I was told by my neurologist that I had fibromyalgia and that the lesions on my brain appeared to be the beginning developments of multiple sclerosis. I was then 38, and I felt that I couldn't possibly live much longer going the way I was going. My mother even told me later that she felt that I might die soon. I was so full of anxiety that I was having trouble swallowing, I was dizzy, and driving long distances would cause me to have panic attacks. I stayed in chronic pain, which couldn't be alleviated. I would go to the doctor and they really couldn't find causes for the pain. I was in bed hours each day with my head hurting so much that my kids were taking care of me."

After thoroughly taking an extensive history and listening to Leanne's story, we began treatment right away. She was placed on a cleansing protocol for her gut and a diet to eliminate common food intolerances. While she experienced withdrawals from popular food items such as donuts and pizza, she found herself feeling excited about meals packed with fruits, vegetables, and lean protein.

"I noticed right away how I was waking up more refreshed, I started having more energy, and the weight started to fall off. My joints felt better, my hands and feet weren't swollen, my headaches became less frequent, my blood pressure came down to the normal range. I started feeling hope again!

Maybe my life wasn't over! How could something as simple as eating a healthy diet and taking one supplement to bring such drastic changes so quickly?

"It is the best feeling in the world to take care of your body and to feel that your body is taking care of you in return. I now experience restful sleep, no anxiety, no migraines, normal blood pressure, no chronic pain, I have lost 50 pounds, and I'm off all prescription medications! I am now nearing nine months of eating healthy. I enjoy all of the vegetables, fruits, meat, nuts, almond milk, almond flour, coconut flour, eggs, and healthy oils that I want. I'm never hungry, my blood sugar is stable, I have constant energy, and I have even started running again just for fun. My precious children are thankful to have their mom back! The changes I have made have even inspired them to eat healthier and exercise more."

With more energy and motivation than she has had in a long time, Leanne urges anyone considering making a change to commit as wholeheartedly as she did.

"If you feel that life is over, please believe me when I say that it is not over! I know what you are feeling, trust me I do. I promise that when you change your diet, your life will change for the better!

Ok, so what specifics can you expect to find in this book?

I have divided the material into three parts of several chapters. In part one, I describe your brain in broad detail, why it's important, what your brain depends on to be healthy and what it needs to function. I also describe what can (and often does) go wrong in Chapter 3 and Chapter 4. Chapter 3 explores what goes wrong in the case of Alzheimer's disease and Parkinson's disease, whilst in Chapter 4 I look at what can go wrong from the perspective of general dementia, and what happens when people suffer from migraines. Both Chapter 3 and Chapter 4 include many useful tips and pieces of practical advice that you can adopt to counteract or prevent these things from happening to you.

In part two of this book, I look at all the natural tools and remedies that have been discovered to scientifically support the brain, heal it, and boost its functions. The tools I describe in part two include amazing natural supplements, the benefits of exercise, sleeping properly, and reducing stress – all the things you can practically use to reclaim your brain. These tools not only deal with the brain directly, but they also support all those factors that the brain depends upon to actually function optimally too.

In part three of this book, I 'bring it all together' and give you a practical and easy to implement plan to follow. This plan contains concrete instructions on supplementation, as well as good simple brain health tips to follow so that you can develop healthy brain habits. I also give actionable advice to follow so that you can actually put all the information covered in parts one and two into practice in your daily life.

I wish you all the best with your health, happiness, and healing. May this book be a huge first step on your journey towards a full and long-lived healthy life – a life filled with smart, wise, and empowering daily choices.

Best Wishes,
Dr. Strong DC, DACNB, CFMP, PAK

I

YOUR AMAZING BRAIN

WHAT IT DOES & WHY IT'S IMPORTANT |THE KEY FACTORS THAT AFFECT YOUR BRAIN | WHAT CAN GO WRONG

1

YOUR BRAIN, YOU, AND YOUR QUALITY OF LIFE

We are incredible beings, capable of creating solutions to seemingly unsolvable problems and achieving great physical feats. At the forefront of our near-infinite possibilities is our control center, our brain, which is involved in just about every activity performed externally, and every single body system internally. Your brain contributes to so much of your life that in many ways it wouldn't be too much of an overstatement to say that you ARE your brain.

Your Brain and You

An important note that you need to understand before we delve into the brain and its connection to health: You do not need to have a degree or a vast understanding of biology to understand the brain. Experts have tried to for centuries and are still learning new things—sometimes even the professionals are completely baffled by certain complex problems in the central nervous system.

Essentially, your brain is made up of four parts: The cerebrum, the cerebellum, the pons, and the medulla oblongata. The cerebrum, housed in the upper part of the brain, is divided into lobes and controls mental state, which includes decision making, regulating emotions, and planning. This part of the brain is one of two parts of the brain that house our gray matter, which regulates our attention, memory, and thoughts in the cerebrum.

The cerebellum is the other part of the brain that houses gray matter. In the cerebellum, gray matter regulates mood, coordination, and precision. The cerebellum itself regulates equilibrium and muscle coordination. The pons is located in front of the cerebellum and essentially serves as a messenger between the cerebrum, cerebellum, and spinal cord. Between the pons and the spinal cord, the medulla oblongata controls more innate responses like breathing, vomiting, and the heartbeat.

Throughout the spinal cord, the brain sends messages to the rest of the body to signal things such as mealtime, when to fall asleep, and whether a sensation should be registered as pain. It also receives messages from the other organs in the body and determines whether to make changes or perform an action. The brain relies on steady blood flow, adequate respiration, and essential nutrients such as water, vitamins, and minerals.

If you take away one thing only from this chapter, it should be that the brain is a powerful but needy organ. To power our bodies at any age and in any state, it needs clean and dependable energy, stimulation, and care. Although it is not a muscle, I strongly advise you to treat it as one. For example, professional athletes follow strict dietary and sleep guidelines to maintain optimal function on their playing fields; however, you do not need to be a professional athlete to prioritize yourself and your body. Research has linked myriad self-care practices, including maintaining a healthy diet and exercise regimen, to sharpening cognitive capabilities. The practices in our book will focus on some of the most common problems.

Why is your brain so Important?

So what is the brain responsible for? What does it do? I would like to suggest the following points as a preliminary answer to these important questions:

Your brain is critically important for, and involved in…

- Your Moods
- Your thinking

- Your memory
- Your muscle movements
- All of your senses
- How you form bonds, attachments, relationships
- How you learn new information
- How you learn new physical skills, and how you ultimately master them
- Your sense of feelings, anxiety, stress, emotions
- Your sleep and wake cycles
- Hunger, drive, physical maturation
- Your sense of self
- And much more...

If you read the above points and stop for a moment to reflect on what this means you will see that your brain is responsible (or at least critically involved in) for almost everything that makes up who you are as an organism. Everything you do, think, feel, learn, say, see, hear, touch, taste, smell, or even dream, relies in some way on your brain functioning properly. So, naturally, we should be concerned with it being healthy, how it works, what affects it, and whether we can support it in some way?

Of course, having a happy healthy brain is a minimum requirement for having a reasonable quality of life, but the more ambitious of you might want to know whether we can do something skillful to help make it function at peak levels.

Others of you reading this might have health conditions linked to your brain, and are looking for a way to heal.

Whatever the case may be for you, whatever the main purpose for your interest is, it stands to reason that knowing a little bit about your brain would be an important and valuable piece of knowledge – something you might be able to actually use to heal yourself, prevent future problems – or perhaps even to optimize the way it functions to enhance a healthy life to new levels of satisfaction and performance. Educating yourself about your brain is the first step to being empowered to affect it positively, and that first step starts here with knowing how important it is.

That is what I want to cover in this first chapter - I want to share information about your brain, how it works, and what factors it relies upon to function. In the next chapter we will look at what can go wrong when one or more of these factors come together, things like poor memory, chronic diseases, migraines, depression, and anxiety. But before we look at problems it is good to know about what affects the brain, what it relies on, to function properly and healthily. After that, you will be in a position to appreciate just why problems can arise. Finally, I'll describe solutions to these problems –easy healthy tips and habits, substances, and activities that will help restore balance to these factors, promote brain health and healing, prevent chronic brain problems, and ultimately boost your brain's performance by giving it the perfect support.

Although the brain is a powerful organ, it relies on us extensively. We experience an extensive amount of wear on our brains throughout the day. Our neurological strength weakens as we age, but illnesses such as dementia, Alzheimer's disease, and Parkinson's disease, should not be an expected consequence of aging. Although we can heal from occasional occurrences, repeated exposures to unhealthy additions can make us suffer in the long term. Poor decisions and adverse exposure, in the long run, can open us up to chronic illnesses that rob us of our vibrancy, memories, and happiness. Ultimately, unhealthy exposure can cut our lives short.

Despite our best efforts, we cannot fully reverse the mental decline that comes with aging. However, we can prevent further cognitive decline from happening and lessen our chance of developing chronic diseases through our lifestyle choices. It is important now more than ever for people to be aware of how their actions impact their bodies because we are living longer than ever before; this opens ourselves up to the possibility of developing illnesses, some of which are currently incurable. Experts believe the number of neurological diagnoses and deaths will rise between now and the year 2050.[1] Consequently, many people will bear the burden of increased medical costs to fend off these diseases and care for those who have already been diagnosed.

Even now, mankind spends billions globally to fend off diseases we could have easily prevented through prioritizing our mental health. In this short chapter, we will briefly describe the key factors that your brain depends on to function properly.

The Key Factors That Influence Brain function

So, what exactly are the key factors that influence how our brain functions? It turns out that the key factors are simple and intuitive provided you keep two main points in mind.

The first point is that the brain needs a lot of energy to work. If you think about it, every time a nerve cell 'sparks' in your brain it releases energy, then the nerve needs to reset and recharge for the next 'spark'. Lots of chemicals are released and absorbed by nerve cells when they are active, so there is a huge demand for these chemicals in an active brain. This is the first point, that the brain needs energy, and anything that impacts the energy supply of the brain will impact how it performs.

The second point to keep in mind is that the brain is a collection of living cells, in a living environment, within a living system. This means that like all living things it requires raw materials, protection, and all the nutrients it might need to function in an optimally healthy way. This second point is related to the first in the sense that energy usually comes from nutrition. But this point is a bit deeper because the brain needs other building block materials to help repair and maintain nerves. The brain relies on the immune system for protection, and it needs an uninterrupted supply of essential nutrients and compounds to help it work properly.

So, given these two main points what might affect the brain's supply of energy, nutrients, and protection?

In short, any of the following would logically have a massive impact:

The Most Direct Factors

Diet & Your Gut Environment

What you eat determines your energy intake, and the kinds of raw materials your body gets to work with – clearly, your brain must be affected by what you eat, as will every other important system or organ in the body like your muscles, skeleton, gut, immune system, heart and blood vessels.

Physical Health

If your body is performing optimally, then the brain is supported properly too – if you have an infection or chronic illness, your brain will be affected along with whatever is currently infected or affected directly.

Damage directly to the brain

Damage to the brain would clearly affect your brain health and functionality.

Your environment

Consider that everything your body becomes exposed to might have an effect on your body's health. Stress, pollution, poisonous pesticides, toxic chemical compounds additives, medicines, and so on – exposure to poison will have powerful effects on your health, and your brain.

Heart & Blood Vessel Health

Your heart and blood vessel health would impact the blood flow to your brain. This is very important because the blood is the way all the energy, nutrients, basic building blocks, oxygen, and immune cells travel to the brain. Waste by-products of a healthy functioning brain also need to be sent away from the brain to other areas of the body for process-ing, recycling, or elimination and removal. A good blood supply, a healthy heart, and unclogged healthy arteries and veins are needed to keep the brain supplied with all it needs and remove the waste it does not want.

All the above makes perfect sense, right? But there are still a few more factors that might not be so obvious just from the two main points above. The reason these might not be as immediately obvious is that they tend to affect the above things indirectly, not directly. A little bit of biological and health-knowledge is necessary for this understanding.

Many of the following factors that I am about to mention next will make sense if you think about them in your own experience of day to day life. The following factors are also critical for brain function and health, albeit a little bit more indirectly than the fundamental factors that I have mentioned already. See if you can recognize them in your own life.

Less Obvious Factors

Sleep

Getting good quality sleep, enough sleep, and regular sleep supports health and brain function in many ways. Poor quality sleep, too much or too little sleep, or irregular sleeping schedules tend to cause disease, ill health, and many other problems; not to mention poor brain performance and health. Just try to remember how difficult it was to think properly and clearly the last time you were sleep-deprived!

Stress & Anxiety

Chronic stress and anxiety tend to cause chemical changes in the body that affect the heart and blood vessels. In addition to that, people under stress often have trouble sleeping which we know affects our brain. People under stress are often pressurized for time and often cope by relying on convenience foods to eat 'on-the-go'. These kinds of foods tend to have poor nutritional content, and often contain pretty toxic additives, sweeteners, colorants, flavor enhancers, and preservatives. Not a good scenario on the food front – and we know diet affects brain health directly and indirectly. The other issue with stress and anxiety is that it drains the body of resources over time because our bodies have to constantly draw on its reserves to cope with demanding and intense situations.[2]

Exercise

I will discuss exercise in more detail throughout this book, but for now, it is important to know that a sedentary lifestyle lacking in exercise has poor outcomes for overall health and terrible consequences for the health of every organ and system within the body. The corollary to this is that being modestly active, engaging in sensible levels of appropriate exercise regularly will confer benefits to your overall health, and support every single organ and system within the body, without exception. Your brain needs exercise, and your brain needs your body to get exercise, especially if it wants to remain healthy, let alone to perform at peak levels.

Neurotransmitter Balance – Having them is not enough, balance is key

These are little messenger molecules that live in the ends of each of our nerve cells. These little messengers are important for our nerves to function properly because they are responsible for bridging the gaps between nerves. In a way, if a nerve wants to send information to its neighbor, then it has to release neurotransmitter messengers to cross the space between those nerve endings. The presence of neurotransmitters lets us control the flow of information in the brain and body. Since nerves conduct information electrically, the body finds a way to control that flow chemically by bridging nerves together or blocking them from speaking to their neighbors. You can think of neurotransmitters as little messenger keys that connect nerves to each other. Without the right amounts of each neurotransmitter in the brain, our brain tends to function in an unbalanced way, leading to many problems like moods, depression, sleep problems, foggy thinking, pain, excitability, memory problems, attention deficits, and many more. These little messengers need to be constantly renewed, recycled, and balanced, they are tiny, part of the nuts-and-bolts chemistry of basic brain function, and they depend on great nutrition, sleep, exercise, and superb nutrients transported by a healthy blood supply to be in balance.

Each one of the factors mentioned above, direct or indirect, are so important for brain health that I will mention them time and time again as we continue throughout this book. Nevertheless, because we are looking closely at your brain's functioning in this first chapter, I think it would be good to take a closer look at neurotransmitters now, in the very next chapter before we move on to other things.

2

A CLOSER LOOK AT NEUROTRANSMITTERS

Neurotransmitters are like tiny keys that enable the body to regulate and control brain activity chemically – they are literally the keys to unlocking your optimal brain function, stable moods, great motivation, reductions in stress, and reductions in anxiety, increase your sense of happiness, and many more.[1]

As we will discover in the next section in this chapter, the messengers in your gut are best optimized by your diet and lifestyle choices – the exact same thing applies here with neurotransmitters in general. This is because the gut and brain are tightly linked, and the common factor linking them is neurotransmitters. What this also means is that your gut health and your brain health are tightly interwoven – they are interdependent.

So, what goes on inside the brain when it's going about its normal activity? It turns out that what goes on inside the brain is tied, ultimately, to neurotransmitters. Even when we are not awake, our brains are working in overdrive to keep us functioning. The unsung heroes of the brain are the billions of messengers regulating our breathing, learning, and everything in between.

Nerve cells, or neurons, in the body have a never-ending mission: they need to send and receive messages throughout the body so it can make the best decisions and act accordingly. However, this mission cannot be conducted alone. At the end of each cell is a synapse or a tiny gap that messages need to pass over. To do their jobs, neurons must be able to convey this message across this tiny space.

This is where we introduce neurotransmitters. These chemicals form after neurons activate and send information into the synapse. The neurotransmitters then respond when those neurons fire and finish the job by sending the message to the other neurotransmitter. Some neurotransmitters can speed up these messages, while others can block the signal from being sent. In short, neurotransmitters are the delivery men for messages between gaps in the brain.

We mentioned that neurotransmitters are chemicals. There are over 60 different kinds of chemicals that serve as couriers between nerve cells. The neurons that help fire the message along are called excitatory neurons and the neurotransmitters linked to this excitation are most commonly acetylcholine, epinephrine, and norepinephrine, and some others.

Consider this; imagine the 'United Parcel Service' (UPS) of chemicals, the core of delivery people who send and deliver messages from your body to the brain's nerve cells and back. The brain, after working hard, depends on its couriers to make sure all its regulatory messages find their way to the right parts of the body.

Neurotransmitters, and the messages they convey, are often hindered by drugs and disease. In the long term, issues with neurotransmitters can result in chronic illnesses such as depression, anxiety, migraines, Alzheimer's, and Parkinson's. While there are so many neurotransmitters that help regulate the body, maintain optimal functioning, and keep everything ticking, it is the following few that I list below that are the main ones implicated in most of the common mental health problems people suffer from today. In most cases, it is not the absence or presence of these neurotransmitters that cause the problem, but rather the unbalanced levels of these neurotransmitters relative to others that seem to be linked with brain problems.

Important Neurotransmitters Linked to Your brain Health

Gamma-aminobutyric Acid (GABA)

GABA regulates motor control, vision, and anxiety levels. This neurotransmitter can promote relaxation and calm which is why pharmaceutical drugs like benzodiazepines are so effective at reducing anxiety – they optimize GABA efficiency in the body. Of course, benzodiazepines have serious and dangerous drawbacks whenever they are used, so I will NOT be recommending them, I only mention them as a way to show how strongly GABA is linked to anxiety levels - there are a whole host of alternatives to pharmaceutical drugs that would achieve better results and health outcomes for you and your brain, particularly in the long run where it matters most – these I will be recommending wholeheartedly when the time comes to share them later n this book.[2]

Dopamine

Dopamine is known for being responsible for pleasurable and rewarding sensations; it's the chemical equivalent to a feel-good response, usually to instant gratification. Indeed, this chemical regulates the coordination of body movements and is commonly known for its role in motivating short-term rewards and addiction.

Acetylcholine

This neurotransmitter is found in both the central and peripheral nervous systems and is most commonly associated with the way our muscles move, i.e. our motor skills. But, Acetylcholine also plays a huge role in learning and memory in addition to muscle movements.

Glutamate

Glutamate plays a role in mental functions like memory and learning. Too much glutamate secretion in the brain leads to over-excitability of the nerves in the brain which tends to wreak havoc on the body. Excesses of this chemical can kill cells, and it is no surprise that glutamate has been linked to Alzheimer's disease, seizures, and strokes. Don't get the wrong idea though, this neurotransmitter is necessary for healthy functioning, just that in excess, the consequences can be disastrous.

Serotonin

Serotonin regulates sleep, sexuality, appetite, mood, and anxiety. A lack of serotonin often results in anxiety disorders such as depression. A fun fact is that your gut contains 90% of your serotonin. So mood disorders such as anxiety and depression may actually stem from your gut.[3]

Epinephrine

This compound basically affects or fuels our 'fight-or-flight' responses in the brain – it is involved in preparing the brain and body for situations that are perceived as extremely challenging and/or dangerous. You may be more familiar with its common name, adrenaline. Epinephrine has a vast number of effects in the body - it regulates blood flow to tissues and other parts of the body when we experience stress, and is a major contributor to cellular damage if levels are chronically high. We need this compound for our heart health, and for alertness, and it is one of the few neurotransmitters that is also a hormone too.

Norepinephrine

Norepinephrine Is the chemical your body is pumping when you experience stress. When your body detects stress, it can release norepinephrine to raise heart rate, release glucose into the blood, and stimulate blood flow. As a neurotransmitter, it can help oversee response time, arousal, and alertness. Low levels of norepinephrine can result in depression or abnormally low blood pressure. Think of Norepinephrine as the chemical neurotransmitter that tells the body, "hey, grab your resources, harness your energy, raise your blood flow, get ready, you need to be on high alert". It is linked to adrenalin but occupies a different stage of the alert response messenger chain.

What Can Go Wrong with Neurotransmitters?

With a system so endlessly complex and so dependent on us for proper functioning, it isn't surprising that things can go wrong. For one, the body can make too much or too little of a particular neurotransmitter. Additionally, enzymes may deactivate too many neurotransmitters, our cells may reabsorb neurotransmitters too quickly.

Occasional damage may explain some of your issues surrounding brain fog, spotty memory, and depression. Neurotransmitter imbalances can create inflammation in the brain, which, as we have discussed, lays waste to the brain's operating capacity. Low levels of glutamate, epinephrine, or norepinephrine can destroy our focus and throw everything into disarray.

A range of causes can be attributed to deficiencies or too many neurotransmitters. However, a plethora of neurological issues can be attributed to neurotransmitter misfiring, including Parkinson's disease and Alzheimer's disease. Even episodic issues with neurotransmitters can impair our memories, cause depression to flare, or create confusion.[4]

Alzheimer's disease has a suggested link to a deficit in acetylcholine, which is essential for processing the memories we make and the lessons we learn. Acetylcholine (ACh) bolsters short-term memory, muscle activation, and arousal. Although not having enough ACh is not the only trait linked to people who suffer from Alzheimer's, a low level is a common characteristic of people who have the disease. Brains suffering from Alzheimer's also often release too much glutamate, which becomes harmful because excessive glutamate secretion eventually overstimulates brain cells causing them to become damaged and die.

It's impossible to fully measure the functioning of your whole brain down to the level of each single nerve cell – that kind of granularity would require technology that is far beyond what we currently have. However, that being said, we do know that supplementing your diet with the appropriate vitamins and nutrients has a beneficial effect in your brain, from the activity of single neurons all the way up to networks of neurons and entire regions of the brain.

In this chapter, we have been exploring the many factors that support brain function – the factors that the brain relies upon to function optimally. One of the main factors underlying all brain function is energy. The brain is energy-hungry, because every time a nerve sparks off and transfers information it uses up a little energy, and there a literally millions upon millions of interconnections between neurons in the brain that have to be working constantly whether awake or asleep, be it day or night, it doesn't matter, they must be constantly in the right balance and cycles so that your brain is happy, and your body stays alive and well.

Speaking of being 'energy-hungry', consider the fact that although the brain constitutes only about 2% of your body weight, it nevertheless accounts for between 20% and 25% of our total energy use daily. So, at a very basic level, our brains need to be fed with what it needs so that it gets enough nutrients, energy, and raw materials to function. Blood supply, diet, oxygenation, energy creation (metabolism), and absence of disease are all important critical factors that need to be addressed to keep the brain functioning optimally.

With all the above factors in mind, we can make a preliminary assessment of certain nutrients and vitamins that would be super beneficial for your brain because they either help the heart and blood vessels, or they keep your energy metabolism balanced, or they protect the delicate nerves in the brain from damage by helping the immune system or mopping up toxic reactive chemicals. The list of nutrients I present very briefly below is a great first step into discovering the kinds of tools you have at your disposal to make a positive difference to your body and brain to eliminate foggy thinking, prevent chronic brain illness, and support peak performance mentally. A first step only because it is from these baseline nutrients that we can go one step further and find food sources that contain them in rich and abundant amounts. Take a look at the list below:

A Preliminary List of Nutrients That Support the Key Factors for your Brain and Your Neurotransmitters

B-Vitamins

Having enough sources of **vitamin B** in our diets is important for metabolizing carbohydrates and fatty acids (energy production). We actually depend on B vitamins to keep our essential operations in check by generating energy in cells and directing that cellular energy in the right direction.

Vitamin B3

This vitamin is also known as niacin, and it is instrumental in fueling other energy sources in our brain. Adequate vitamin B3 sources in our brain stimulate dopamine (an important neurotransmitter related to pleasure, motivation, and the feeling of satisfaction or reward) production in our brains and produce chemicals that are instrumental in energy production.

A lack of vitamin B3 can lead to neurological issues including dementia, fatigue, delusional thinking, lack of focus, and shortness of breath. Vitamin B3 can be found in eggs, rice, turkey, fish, beef, chicken, and legumes. So, increasing these foods will ensure that you get enough dietary vitamin B3 provided the sources are organic, healthy, and free of toxic chemicals and pathogens. If you need a boost, turn to these fat and protein-rich options.

Vitamin B5 ("pantothenic acid")

This vitamin helps us to metabolize sugar and fatty acids. When your body uses this vitamin to produce the neurotransmitter acetylcholine we experience better energy levels during the day, reduced stress, better functioning immune systems, healthier-looking skin and hair (anti-aging), and better regulation of important parts of our nervous system (autonomic nervous system). Like most other B-vitamins, B5 is most commonly found in meats, but you can get in bananas, avocados, sunflower seeds, and spinach too.

Iron

Iron is vital for most facets of our bodies. Iron deficiencies during pregnancy and childhood can lead to serious developmental issues. It just so happens that, oftentimes, we do not get enough iron in our diets. However, we need enough iron in our diet to make neurotransmitters like serotonin, dopamine, and norepinephrine. We also need it to recycle these neurotransmitters after their jobs are completed. Iron is found in meat, seafood, spinach, legumes, pumpkin seeds, quinoa, broccoli, tofu, and dark chocolate (very dark chocolate).

Magnesium (Mg)

Mg is important for hundreds of chemical reactions in the body related to brain functions. Too little magnesium can result in neurological issues including muscle spasms and tremors. This deficiency has also been linked to Epilepsy, Alzheimer's, Parkinson's, chronic pain, and migraines. Magnesium helps muscles contract (including heart muscles), regulate blood pressure, metabolize insulin, and create essential proteins for the body. Too little magnesium can spell terror for the cells in our body. Consider that as many as 95% of those who suffer from magnesium deficiency may also suffer from attention deficit hyperactivity disorder (ADHD).

A good way to ensure you are receiving enough magnesium is to eat magnesium-rich foods like leafy green vegetables (as well as cruciferous veggies), avocados, bananas, and beans. Getting these critical nutrients from our food is very important if you want a healthy high functioning super-optimized brain, but, the problem with relying solely on dietary sources for these nutrients is that our bodies have a lot to contend with in modern life. Stress, anxiety, environmental pollutants, and convenience foods which are poor in nutritional content – this is not even mentioning infection, inflammation, disease, and many more.

The body is not really very good at absorbing high quantities of these nutrients from our food, so if we become deficient in any of these nutrients because of the stresses that leech the body of these compounds we may never catch up to healthy levels. This is why supplementing with these compounds makes complete sense, especially in the modern context of a hectic and busy urban life.

Other Nutrients and Compounds Important for Neurotransmitters in the brain

Iodine

Iodine regulates growth, reproduction, metabolism, and cell development. A lack of iodine can result in intellectual impairment and developmental issues. Iodine is also very important when it comes to regulating thyroid health. Iodine deficiency is one of the most common, yet most preventable causes of cognitive issues in the body. Foods that include a good amount of iodine include seaweed, cod, dairy products, tuna, shrimp, prunes, eggs, and lima beans.

Calcium

Calcium is well known as the mineral essential for healthy bones. However, it is also responsible for regulating gene expressions and cognitive function. It helps the neurons fire off messages and gets the whole process started. Some studies have linked calcium deficiency to increased cognitive decline. You can find calcium for your diet by eating broccoli, cheese, chia seeds, celery, legumes, almonds, leafy greens, whey, rhubarb, milk, edamame, tofu, and figs.

Omega-3 fatty acids

Omega-3's can go a long way in helping fatty acids EPA and DHA keep everything running as usual in the brain. These two chemicals have been shown to help to develop brains. We can help our brain by promoting these building blocks of the chemical balances in the brain. Omega-3 fatty acids are found in foods including fish, fish oil, walnuts, chia seeds, flaxseed, soybeans, and soybean oil. However, we are not great at converting the energy from these foods, using a fish oil supplement may be the best way of ensuring your brain is receiving these critical nutrients.

Serotonin

Serotonin is actually a neurotransmitter, one of the most important ones for having balanced moods and being happy. Proper levels of serotonin help us to feel energized and generally happier, without it we feel drained, foggy in the head, depressed, and often have trouble sleeping. The surprising thing about serotonin is that we can get it directly from some food sources – tasty sources include kiwis, bananas, eggs, walnuts, and turkey.

Your neurotransmitters are the little chemicals that allow the body to control the way nerves talk to each other, they have countless important tasks to perform and depletion in any one of them will cause your brain to function poorly with serious potential effects on your quality of life. Making sure your body has everything it needs to make its neurotransmitters is like making sure it can do its job at a chemical level and these building blocks must come from your diet and supplementation. Vitamins and minerals are essential for your neurotransmitter profile, and I have mentioned the most important ones that you should focus on to make sure that they stay in a good balanced supply. Remember that an inability to absorb these nutrients can lead to a decrease in neurotransmitters and thus lead to chronic illness, depression, and a wide variety of very serious unhealthy body states – supplementation can be key, especially when the diet doesn't cut it.

Neurotransmitter Brain Tip #1:

By educating yourself and understanding what leads to cognitive issues, you can prevent these symptoms from occurring and avoid chronic issues. You can't necessarily prevent the onset of these diseases, but you will be able to greatly delay their onsets.

Neurotransmitter Brain Tip #2:

The brain controls nearly every bodily function. If it is impaired, other parts of the body will be as well. So, treat your brain right; feed it the nutrients that it requires and aid in its cognitive functioning by mentally training it and "keeping it in shape."

Speaking of diet affecting neurotransmitters, the brain, and moods, there are actually a few beneficial kinds of foods and food groups that will not only benefit your neurotransmitters but also enhance the health of your gut too.

The gut and the brain are closely linked, if your gut is out of balance, then your brain will be too. This is a very important factor in your brain health and it turns out that what you eat affects what you think and how you feel.

In fact, the link between the gut, diet, and brain function is so important that I have devoted the whole of Chapter 4 to it. For now, however, I just want to mention that certain food groups are beneficial to your neurotransmitters – a fact that will also be shown to be important for gut health later on in this book. Some of these important foods and food groups are:

- Legumes
- Lean meat and alternative protein, such as tofu
- Leafy green vegetables
- Fruits
- Fermented foods
- Other high-fiber vegetables (no grains; and they

must be gluten-free)

Making sure to load your diet with the above foods and groups will have massive benefits for your brain and I will share more on this later. A great way to eat more of these foods is to put some of them into smoothies, and in the final sections of this book, I have given some example smoothies for you to try for yourself. Delicious, healthy, easy, natural, energizing through the day, and most importantly, brain-boosting!

Smoothies are a great way to 'sneak' these foods into your diet whilst reducing empty calories and boosting brain function. For example, you can try putting some greens into a smoothie or health shake, or substituting one of your meaty entrees at dinner times for a spinach-mushroom mix. You may find that you feel full after eating much more protein and vegetable fibers with only fractions of the unhealthy fat and cholesterol from meat. Eating fewer calories while having the same nutrient content in your food is one open secret to extending your life-span, improving your brain function, and living a healthier happier life.

Diet and Exercise: You (and Your Brain) are What You Eat!

In chapter 4 I discuss eating for your happiness, your brain, and your mood, and in one of the last chapters of this book, I discuss exercise. However, I feel it is worth mentioning something about these two factors here just to give you the idea so that you keep it in mind as you move forward.

There's a reason why many people buy into the generalization that Americans are often overweight and unhealthy. Basically, for a huge number of American citizens it is, in short, true — Not to say that only Americans are like this, but that for many, the perception is that this is more common for American's nowadays than people from other countries. Why would this possibly be the case? I contend that it has everything to do with the current entrenched cultural approaches we Americans have to our eating habits, nutrition, and lifestyles.

So, when it comes to eating in the United States, what typically comes to mind? In many cases, the foods that are easiest to get and cheapest to purchase, tend to contain red meat, saturated fat, excessive amounts of sugar, and artificial additives like colorants, preservatives, and flavor enhancers. In the 'States' it often seems that quantity trumps quality – value is defined by how much I get for how little I have to do or pay – convenience and taste and price will tend to trump actual value in the form of nutrition and health – expedience and profiteering are the key factors for producers, convenience and ease are the key factors for consumers.

The consequence of this mindset towards food has opened the gateway to a gradual cultural preference for foods that have way too much sugar, salt, and preservatives prepackaged for takeout, or microwaved in seconds. We don't have much money or time these days, so such foods are extremely tempting, and tasty – over time we have learned to really crave these foods, and feel satisfied when we eat them. But, what happens in our body when all we feed it is nutrient-poor fat, sugar, low-grade meat, and synthetic chemicals? - A health disaster of epic proportions with an explosion of chronic degenerative lifestyle diseases. Our brains suffer for it too, so, it has to stop. Time to make some different choices, time to be smart...do your mind and body a favor, give them what they need and thrive on; then see how much you enjoy life.

There are actually many healthy food sources available everywhere in the U.S., it isn't that there is a lack of options. The main issue has to do with the *approach* to food. In other countries, fresh, organic ingredients take precedence over artificial sweeteners and preservatives, and people slow down to enjoy what they are eating. Indeed, many countries view clean, healthy eating as a pleasure rather than an obligation. Other countries also eat considerably less than we do. In reality, many U.S. residents could cut down their daily caloric intake by as much as half. Our attitudes towards portion size have been formed by working long hours on farms engaging in extensive physical activity. That is not as much the case now, as many of us are sedentary.

Our culture towards food and portion size aside, eating poorly is too dangerous to sustain. Nearly one in three adults in the United States are clinically overweight according to the World Health Organization; consequently, they are open to cardiovascular illnesses, vitamin deficiencies, and organ failure in the future. These health concerns, ranging from high blood pressure to heart attacks, kidney failure, and brittle bones, place stress on the brain to work harder or compensate for these issues. For instance, our brain depends on blood flow and oxygen. The brain is thus jeopardized by poor cardiovascular health.

Next, we can focus on consuming a wide variety of healthy foods to keep our strength and ensure our nutritional needs are met. Research has suggested we can curb our chance of developing neurodegenerative diseases by focusing on our consumption of fruits, vegetables, and nuts, as well as cutting down our caloric intake. The positive consequences of changing our diet are bountiful. Observing a healthier diet translates to lower blood pressure, weight loss, lower cholesterol levels, and more energy.

Finally, healthy eating will help you muster up all the energy you need for a successful day filled with mental stimulation and exercise.

So, healthy eating and exercise come together to complement each other are two lifestyle factors that are critical to your health in general, and to your brain in particular – especially in the long run which is precisely where people start to get major chronic brain illnesses (we'll look at these in Chapter 3 – where things go wrong).

Home, history, genes, and Environment

As humans, we grow and change throughout our lives. This is true not only for us as psychological beings, 'people', but in many ways, our bodies exhibit the same characteristic too. Our bodies are also constantly changing and dynamically adapting to their environment and experiences – something that was true for you even before you were born.

A lot of our evolution and development is linked to our genetics, but our genes don't determine everything, far from it. Many people with specific disease-causing genes ever go on to express any negative symptoms associated with those genes. In reality, many of the genes we do inherit only ever express in our body and health given the right environmental triggers. The actions of our parents and the places where we grow up can have a profound effect on our long-term health in terms of exposure, and learning – learned behavior in terms of coping with stress, problem-solving, relationships, and eating behavior radically affect our health throughout an entire lifetime.

Consider that it is also true that people are born to different socio-economic contexts with different levels of access to infrastructure, healthcare, education, and cultural patterns of eating, resting, sleeping, and working. Many places in the U.S. do not have access to clean drinking water. Polluted city environments can often make breathing difficult, especially for people with pre-existing health concerns and problems. In cities across the United States, grocery stores offering fresh fruits and vegetables are sometimes inaccessible, if not entirely nonexistent.

Everyone's upbringing and daily life look different; however, income inequality and inherently unequal housing standards can place many people in less than desirable environments – dangerous criminal presence, pollutants, and for many a noticeable and regrettable lack of common community green spaces, clean waterways, and fresh clean breathable air.

We are also beholden to the behaviors of our parents, starting from conception. It is common knowledge that the consumption of alcohol, tobacco, caffeine, or other substances will result in illness and lifelong developmental issues. People who do not understand this risk may be more likely to expose their kids to the same risk; the same people who are more likely to live in areas laden with environmental toxins may also inadvertently expose them to risk, as well.

After birth, home life will also have a profound effect on all facets of our health. Family issues can also form our responses to stress and affect our relationship with the world. People who have grown up with strained family life could have an increased risk of forming an unhealthy relationship with food, drugs, or alcohol, and even other people. One thing is certain though, taking care of the environment and circumstances in which you find yourself, eating good food, developing healthy lifestyle habits, looking after your body, and keeping your brain in balance all work synergistically together to increase your overall quality of life. A happy brain means a happy you, with good energy, and sharp learning – this naturally leads to spill-over effects in other areas of life like the people we meet job success, family relationships, and every other facet of life. Doing 'good' for your brain means doing good for others too, it makes complete sense once you think about it.

What to Remember from Chapter 1 and Chapter 2

I have shared a lot of information with you in the first two chapters of this book, and if you feel it might be overwhelming at this point, then don't worry. The main idea that you should take from the information we have covered so far is that the brain is important for everything that matters. Not only that, but the way that we live, what we choose to eat, how we exercise, how we use our brains, and how we approach our environment all affect our brains.

The brain relies on key factors to function properly, these are:

- Good energy supply - metabolism needs to be in balance.
- A steady supply of nutrients so that it can use and recycle neurotransmitters.
- Lots of oxygen
- A healthy non-toxic brain tissue environment.

If you think about these three things carefully then you realize that anything you do that affects these four things will impact the health and functioning of your brain. What kinds of things could affect the above things? The main factors that you can control or influence positively to affect brain health in your favor include:

- Diet (for energy and nutrients, and a happy gut leading to a happy brain)
- Heart and blood vessel health
- to supply the brain with nutrients, energy, and oxygen
- to remove the toxic build-up of compounds that

might accumulate in the brain through normal functioning

- A healthy Immune system
- Prevent and fight infection
- Stress-free lifestyle, good sleep, good exercise
- No exposure to toxic chemicals that might cause damage.
- Neurotransmitters! These tiny little chemical messengers are extremely important to your brain and body. They need to be in correct balance, and your body needs the raw materials to make them replenish their numbers when things get depleted.

The above things are the kinds of things that promote brain function because they make sure that your heart and blood vessels feed the brain with enough of what it needs. Your diet makes sure that the things the brain needs are actually available in the body for the blood to transport it.

Stress and sleep affect the way the brain functions, and both stress and sleep are linked to poor choices, foggy thinking, and the generation of toxic chemicals in the body that can be detrimental to health.

Eating well supports a healthy immune system, and reduces toxic by-products from breaking down your food which helps protect the brain from becoming inflamed and damaged over time. Exercise is massively supportive of overall health too and will oxygenate the brain and protect its fragile cells from being vulnerable to infection, inflammation, and poor health too.

All of the above factors can affect our neurotransmitter levels, but eating properly, exercising, sleeping properly, and reducing stress all help the gut to be happy, which also helps the brain to have good neurotransmitter levels.

That's all you need to remember from the first two chapters. These are the main points that I will time and again emphasize throughout the rest of the book.

In the next chapter, I will look at what can go wrong with the brain in cases of chronic illness or common neurological problems like migraines and foggy thinking. The aim of the next chapter is not to make you into an expert on these diseases and conditions, but rather to show you that in each case of serious chronic illness it is time and time again our lifestyle and diet that contribute to making the brain a toxic organ – resulting in a diagnosable disease later in life.

Each one of the problems I share with you in the next chapter, like Alzheimer's disease(AD), Parkinson's disease (PD), migraines, foggy thinking, multiple sclerosis, and others, tend to be caused by the same underlying mechanisms – damage to the brain because of inflammation.

The unique mechanism by which this inflammation comes about and eventually becomes too much for the body to fix might be different in each case, but usually, it is our diet and lifestyle choices, combined with our environmental exposure and genetics that gradually, day by day over many years, lead to some kind of chronic degenerative problem or diagnosable illness.

Migraines and foggy thinking are just early signs of problems that are sure to come later – if nothing is done to change your health.

As for what makes brains perform poorly and become ill? That almost always has to do with inflammation, and how our chronically poor health choices unbalance the factors lead to inflamed tissues and systems.

How do our daily health choices end up unbalancing the key factors that I introduced in this chapter to eventually cause problems? It is quite simple, if you don't look after the important things we talked about in this chapter, you'll eventually get the problems I will soon share with you in the next chapter. The question is, how do you look after the things we talked about in this chapter? The answer to that will come throughout this book as we explore the issue together. For now, let's dive into what goes wrong, just so that we can see how in each case it is the same or similar underlying things that give rise to brain and body problems over time.

3

WHEN THINGS GO WRONG (A)
(ALZHEIMER'S DISEASE AND PARKINSON'S DISEASE)

Common Neurological Problems

When the brain is not operating at its best, it becomes susceptible to minor health concerns at best and chronic diseases at worst. I have compiled a list of the most common neurological problems faced by people I've treated; most of these issues have longer chapters dedicated to explaining and treating them. Before you begin treatment, please see a certified physician for diagnosis and consult with a functional medicine practitioner before starting a routine.

Memory Issues

Do you find yourself forgetting simple facts or blanking on things you shouldn't? For most people, it is normally a mere irritation, where for others it can be a more concerning symptom. Memory issues are among the most common symptoms of cognitive dysfunction. Thus, we can attribute multiple potential factors to foggy memory; among the most common are depression and anxiety, as well as the medical treatments used to offset these mental health issues. Our memory may also be affected by our consumption of alcohol or illicit drugs, external stress, and poor sleep quality.

Although there are medical issues that can cause memory issues, there are also benign factors that can cause them too. External stressors that can affect a person's memory can influence any person and at any age. Memory issues also affect younger populations, particularly in college students. Young people in their early 20s tend to pull all-nighters to study, but this can have a noticeable effect on their memory consolidation. Sleep is needed to consolidate any short-term memories from the frontal lobe that have been made during the day into longer-term memories in the hippocampus. This is also why cramming the night before an exam is an ineffective way to retain information – sleep deprivation due to being up all night will radically impair your ability to fix your memories into your long term store, as well as impair your ability to retrieve information that has already been stored successfully.

Multiple factors can precipitate memory loss. Some causes may be benign, while others may have more ominous causes. The brain will always be a complex organ that allows for higher-order functioning in human beings and may be difficult to understand. But, there are certain factors that you can personally look out for and take action against if you are concerned about potentially dangerous outcomes.

Migraines

An all-too-common effect after stress, sudden dietary or sleep changes, or bright lights, is a throbbing headache that takes away whole days from our work, leisure, and family time. Everyone is different when it comes to the migraines they experience and their exact causes. Many people experience the same symptoms, which are pulsating pain on one side of the head, vomiting, exhaustion, disorientation, and loss of balance.

There are other causes of very severe headaches, and many of them can be just as debilitating as migraines. If you do struggle with headaches, it is important to monitor what your triggers are, because some headaches are precipitated by different causes. There are several reasons that one can develop migraines, but these are normally only limited to one or two per person. It is, generally, highly improbable that a person would have more than two precipitating causes of their migraines.

Some of the most common reasons why you might have a migraine can be:[1] [2] [3]

- Too much or too little sleep
- Caffeine withdrawal after continuous excessive intake
- Consumption of foods containing preservatives and artificial substances such as MSG (monosodium glutamate), nitrates, sulfates, tyramine, or aspartame
- Skipping meals
- Overwhelmed senses from bright lights, overpowering smells, or loud noises
- Hormonal changes
- Stress and anxiety

Brain Fog

Brain fog is exactly what it sounds like: a cloud of confusion that can result in sluggishness, confusion, and delayed responses. Brain fog can result from sleep deprivation, depression, or consuming too much sugar. Additionally, people may experience brain fog if they fail to establish routines such as a consistent bedtime and morning call.

This type of problem can be very irritating and debilitating for people that are trying to cope in high-stress environments. One of the best ways to combat the feeling of a sluggish foggy brain is to sufficiently hydrate and get moving. Cardiovascular exercise increases oxygenation to the cerebral tissue and makes your brain feel much clearer. Keep in mind that your brain also needs adequate hydration to function optimally; sometimes just having a glass of water or two will help clear up any foggy feelings that you may have.

Anxiety and Depression

Anxiety disorders are among the most common mental health issues affecting people globally. Anxiety and depression can affect all of us at any point in our lives, particularly in stressful situations or following traumatizing events. Part of this is the body's way of protecting us from harm. However, for others, anxiety and depression are daily struggles that can affect sleep patterns, sex drive, appetite, and social lives.[4]

Anxiety and depression may be commonly seen, but they are very serious mental health problems that have led to thousands of suicides in the past decade; research has found that more than 70% of people that attempt suicide struggle with mental health problems like anxiety or depression.[5] [6]

These types of mental health disorders can affect anyone. They do not discriminate based on race, gender, social standing, or popularity. Two tragic examples of these types of disorders were when the world mourned the loss of both the famous actor, Robin Williams, and the band Linkin Park's lead vocalist, Chester Bennington because they struggled with depression and other mental health issues. There are thousands of other examples of suicide and self-harm that can be attributed to anxiety and depression. These mental health issues need to be taken as seriously as any other medical condition and treated accordingly. Fortunately, there are both medical and natural ways that these disorders can be treated and alleviated. [7] [8]

Chronic Illnesses

All of the aforementioned neurological problems have a few factors in common that people should keep in mind when wanting to treat these problems naturally. People who experience them may not have structured habits, nutritious diets, stress management skills, or tools to help them cope with rapidly changing situations.

These illnesses may be a hindrance, at best, to our daily lives. However, if left unchecked, they can lay waste to our cognitive abilities and spell trouble for us later in life. Many of the chronic illnesses we discuss in this book begin naturally as a mixture of symptoms that gradually become worse. Many of these diseases are incurable, but with the right supplements and diet, they can be managed. In many cases, it is only with a mix of the two that we can see an improvement.

Alzheimer's disease (AD)

Alzheimer's disease is, unfortunately, an irreversible disorder that slowly destroys the thinking skills and memory capabilities developed throughout life; often involving serious memory impairment, personality changes and ultimately leading to the death of the individual. [9] [10]

At present, a cure for AD has not been found; however, research has uncovered a large body of information on the functional and structural changes in the brain seen during AD progression as well as a lot of statistical population data linked to this disorder. At the moment, the data suggests that the biggest risk factor for AD is age – the older you are, the more likely it is for you to develop AD. This particular disease most commonly affects people in their mid-60s, although research has found that early-onset Alzheimer's (of the genetic variants) can affect people as early as their 30s, and in extreme cases can often emerge at even younger ages. [11]

To make it clear, studies have found that cases of AD have increased alongside the increase in the prevalence of aging populations - this trend is seemingly set to continue with one study estimating a possible 16 million cases of diagnosed AD in populations over the age of 65 years by 2050. [12]

What typically happens in Alzheimer's disease?

This disease is characterized by the slow disconnection of the brain's nerve cells and neural connections in the brain. That activity within the brain translates to the slow unraveling of memories and the loss of patient agency. The most advanced stages of Alzheimer's leave people unable to take care of themselves and can render people confused, agitated, and combative. Alzheimer's is the most common cause of dementia. Aside from memory loss, symptoms of Alzheimer's include changes in planning or problem-solving, confusion with time, difficulty understanding visual images, trouble speaking or writing, poor judgment, withdrawal from work or social activities, difficulty completing familiar tasks, and changes in mood.

In severe cases of Alzheimer's disease, people tend to pass away because their brains "forget" how to function adequately. This means that they ultimately die because their brains can't function on basic levels any longer. Basic functions like breathing and swallowing can ultimately become affected and stop functioning.

Parkinson's disease[13]

Parkinson's disease comes in many shapes and forms. It seems to be more common in men and older people and affects 20 out of 1,000 people over the age of 70.

However, most instances of Parkinson's disease are the cause of damaged brain nerve cells, damaged neural pathways, and the damaged capacity to regulate dopamine. People with Parkinson's may eventually suffer from a lack of balance or constantly rigid muscles. Parkinson's symptoms include hunching over or stooping, dizziness, fainting, a soft or low voice, constipation, trouble moving, sleep issues, small handwriting, loss of smell, and tremors.

There are varying degrees in the severity of Parkinson's diseases, and although a healthy lifestyle may not be able to cure this type of debilitating illness, it will definitely slow down its progression and slow down the onset of symptoms.[14]

Some Good Advice for Handling Chronic Illnesses In General

It may seem inevitable that, eventually, our cognitive health will decline and we will open ourselves up to these types of cruel illnesses. However, researchers have made great strides in better understanding our brains' needs and the direct impact of our choices on our long-term cognitive health.

For instance, we know now that while these illnesses predominantly affect people in their 50s, symptoms can arise in people in their early adulthood years in severe cases. Experts have pointed to early signs of mental decline and have noted signs and symptoms that one should be cognizant of.

In what experts call Age-Associated Memory Impairment (AAMI), they have pinpointed some predecessors and precipitating factors that can show signs of Alzheimer's—complaints of trouble recalling memories and becoming unusually and combatively confused will translate to progressively worsening scores on analysis tests. Some 40% of people aged 50-59 suffer from this. The likelihood of people that suffer from this impairment increases by 10% for each succeeding decade.

As these illnesses can begin manifesting in earlier years, it means there is no time like the present to work on undoing years of disarray.

We need to remember that we should preserve our head-space and listen to our bodies. This includes our physical, mental, and emotional health. Mindfulness goes a long way to making us feel right and will help us act our best. Taking stock of our feelings helps ward off anxiety or depression, and simply makes us feel younger. By challenging our minds to focus on the present instead of dwelling on the past, we naturally force our minds to slow down and become aware of the swirling thoughts inside our minds.

Carve some time out of your day to practice mindfulness. It will ultimately be beneficial to you.

Strong Brain Tips:

- By educating yourself and understanding what leads to cognitive issues, you can prevent these symptoms from occurring and avoid chronic issues.

- We tend to imagine our brain as this foreign, untouchable, self-moderating thing that remains unaffected by our actions or activities. However, this isn't completely true. Your brain does regulate itself, and it even functions while you are asleep, but that doesn't mean that it is unaffected by your conscious waking activities. You can (must) do your part to keep it operating optimally. If your health is compromised, then your brain will be affected negatively because its health and functioning heavily depends on the health and functioning of other bodily systems.

If you look after your health and the health of your brain, then you will help to slow any potential onsets of these types of illnesses.

Alzheimer's disease & Its Link to Lifestyle Choices[15]

Alzheimer's disease (AD) is the most prevalent neurodegenerative disease of our time, as well as one of the most common causes of death in older populations with no known cure. More than 600,000 died from the disease in 2010, and that number is expected to nearly triple by 2050 when experts believe that approximately 1.6 million will die from AD-related problems. Alzheimer's disease often comes about over years, even decades, and is most likely to affect people over 65 years old. It is generally a slow-developing cognitive illness. As our life expectancy increases, more people will have to factor in getting this disease, or will they?

Symptoms of Alzheimer's may be more noticeable from loved ones and friends' perspectives than your own. An often-missed sign is forgetting newly learned information because Alzheimer's begins in the region of the brain that affects learning. As the disease progresses, it makes people confused and disoriented about their belongings. In the long term, the disease causes serious memory loss, thus causing people to forget time, place, and year; grow suspicious about family and friends; and lose the ability to swallow, speak, or walk.

Experts are still perplexed about exactly where Alzheimer's starts. However, they do know this: this disease damages and kills neurons. If you recall in chapter 3 in our discussion of neurotransmitters, you'll recall that the brain is a complex network of cells, proteins, and membranes. In the case of Alzheimer's, protein fragments (called "plaques") build up between cells, while twisted protein fibers build up in cells and tangle. Everyone develops these tangles and plaque build-up; however, Alzheimer's patients tend to build these at a far higher rate than people without the disease, and these abnormalities spread from crucial parts of the brain to all other regions. The cause of this is unknown and so is the effect on the brain before the cells die off. When they do, it's that destruction of nerve cells that leads to the slow-but-deadly escalation of symptoms.

There's no doubt that this disease is horrible. It is not only painful for people to realize they are losing their memories, experiences, and joys that make them human; it is just as painful for the friends and family who watch helplessly as their loved ones slip away. Alzheimer's should not be considered a normal process of aging. Treating Alzheimer's through traditional means costs nearly $28,000 per year. That said, no survey can account for how much is lost for patients as a whole.

What Causes Alzheimer's?

Experts are not precisely sure of a single factor that causes Alzheimer's. However, a lot of factors can contribute to people's likelihood of developing the disease, and there are ways to both minimize your chance of developing it, reverse symptoms, and mitigate the disease's progression.

Alzheimer's may affect hundreds of thousands of people, but it really isn't well understood. But, what is well understood about this disease is how to slow its progression.

Age

Age is the greatest risk factor for developing dementia and Alzheimer's. The chance of developing Alzheimer's doubles every five years after a person reaches 65 years old. By 85 years of age, the risk of developing Alzheimer's disease increases by almost one-third.[16]

Since we understand that this disease has a higher prevalence in older populations, anyone over the age of 60 must go for regular cognitive checkups to ensure that they are still healthy mentally. Also, start treating any symptoms as soon as they begin, because early prevention is your best defense against this debilitating disease.

Previous Injuries

Head injuries may increase your risk of one-day developing dementia. Serious injuries, especially as you grow older, may make you more likely to develop the disease. Head injuries, as well as repetitive injuries to the spinal cord and brain, can result in more serious developments in cognitive diseases later on in life. A stellar example of this is shown in the Will Smith movie "Concussion," which shows how quickly cognitive diseases can affect football players that sustain repetitive head injuries.

To protect yourself (and your brain) from future issues, take good care of yourself by minimizing potential harm to yourself or your head. Wear a helmet whenever participating in contact sports, riding motorcycles or bicycles, or operating dangerous machinery. As you age, consider implementing guardrails, softer flooring, or special accommodations to prevent any chance of injury. Although accidents are going to happen, your mental clarity is worth the extra money or the extra five seconds of precaution. Ultimately, equipping yourself with some of these provisions is almost certain to be cheaper than treating Alzheimer's.

Family History

Although having a relative who suffers from Alzheimer's may seem like developing the disease is inevitable, very few Alzheimer's cases stem from a genetic predisposition towards the disease. However, it does raise your likelihood of developing the disease.

It has normally been found that people who experience cognitive impairment from Alzheimer's disease stemming from a genetic link will most likely experience it much earlier in life. It becomes even more likely that if you have a parent or sibling who has Alzheimer's, you may be more predisposed to develop the disease. The more people you have in your direct family who develop the disease, the more likely it is that you may also develop it yourself.

When it comes to genetic propensities towards Alzheimer's, some genes can contribute to our risk and genes that basically promise the disease will occur in you. "Risk genes" increase the odds you will develop Alzheimer's without guaranteeing you will develop it. Several different genes can increase the odds of developing Alzheimer's. "Deterministic genes" are extremely rare, but basically guarantee whoever holds them will develop the disease. If you know of any cases of Alzheimer's in your family, consider taking a DNA test for the disease. Doing so will give you peace of mind and maybe give you clarity on the odds at hand. It can also prepare to take proper steps to ensure you have the highest quality of life.

Unless you have the extremely rare gene that guarantees the development of the disease, the odds of you developing Alzheimer's are relatively low. Genetics may raise your likelihood, but they don't have to be a prognosis. As you'll see in the next sections, there are actions you can do and steps you can take to mitigate your risk of developing the disease. The idea is to take action before the disease progresses to an irreversible state. It is important to take any claims of genetic determinism, or 'inevitability', with a grain of salt. Not only do you inherit your genes you're your family, but you also inherit your diet, lifestyle choices, and the environment that your family finds itself in. Those external factors (sometimes called "epigenetic factors") are much more critical when it comes to evaluating your risks for AD because those factors are what ultimately determine whether your genetic vulnerabilities actually express themselves – not everyone with genes for some chronic illness actually goes on to develop an illness, it takes more than just your genes.

Another Hollywood example of this type of familial link to Alzheimer's comes about in Julianne Moore's example in "Still Alice." This movie dives into the possibilities of developing early-onset Alzheimer's because of genetic links. It may be a difficult movie to watch, but it does help one understand the full effects of this cognitive illness.

Diet and Health

I cannot stress enough how intrinsically related the brain is to the plethora of choices we are tasked with making daily. The sum of our decisions can dictate whether we one-day experience trouble with our hearts, blood pressure, cholesterol levels, and cognitive function. Alzheimer's is also known as Type 3 Diabetes due to the inflammatory effect sugar has on the brain leading to cognitive decline.

Our brains cannot operate without a steady and reliable source of blood pumped by a strong cardiopulmonary system. By eating unhealthy food and neglecting self-care, you are opening yourself to the possibility of hypertension, stroke, heart attack, diabetes, and heart disease — all of which may easily pave the way to developing Alzheimer's. Research has suggested that people who suffer from strokes may experience more plaque and twists in the brain.

Unhealthy decisions add up over time leading to an increased risk for chronic disease. Much like nicotine, foods high in sugar, salt, and other additives are a lot easier to ingest and keep returning to than healthy foods. Much like smoking, high fructose or sodium items will not produce the same effect on your brain over time, requiring you to eat more for that same dopamine response. There are multiple ways of bad habits, over time, can increase our likelihood of developing Alzheimer's. For one, eating these unhealthy foods can create oxidative stress in your brain, which can also lead to inflammation in the brain. Poor food choices can also, over time, cause your brain-gut axis to break down. The breakdown of the brain-gut axis may result in a faster aging process in the brain, thus causing cells to die off at a quicker pace.

The western diet remains a major threat to our health and cognitive awareness. Not only are we eating nutrient-poor foods that are rich in fat, sugar, salt, and preservatives, but we are eating far too much of them. Because those foods are not nutritious, but rather addictive and unsubstantial.[17]

Researchers with the U.S. government have recommended a diet rich in whole foods, lean protein, and fewer calories. The Dietary Approaches to Stop Hypertension (DASH) utilizes the power of plant-based nutrition to battle Alzheimer's and other forms of dementia. Its portions of food per week may resemble the food pyramid. However, instead of five or six food groups, the instructions recommend you take in nutrients from 10 different groups.

DASH Diet Recommendations:

- Six servings per week of leafy green vegetables
- One serving per day of other vegetables
- Two servings per week of berries
- One serving of fish per week
- Three servings of beans per week
- Five servings per week of nuts
- Two servings of chicken or turkey per week
- Olive oil at most meals (try best to keep from heating)
- Alcohol and other substances in moderation

The inclusion of these basic food alterations can greatly improve a person's cognitive symptoms and can help reduce the development of any cognitive diseases. The DASH diet is also known as the Mediterranean diet; the plan models European portion sizes and emphasis on fresh food. For many Europeans, eating well and eating whole foods is a pleasure, not a health obligation. It is for this reason among many others that overall health overseas is better than it is in the United States.

Scientists are not certain why the Mediterranean diet helps ward off dementia and whether a proper diet can quell the likelihood of developing Alzheimer's. The current school of thought is that maintaining good cardiovascular health may in turn help maintain brain health. Experts also believe the diet may slow down toxins from entering the brain. Whatever the reason, we could all do well to critically assess the foods we put into our bodies and rediscover the joy of taking back some control from the plagues of society. If you are interested in taking a permanent and positive step towards boosting your mental health, consider starting small by eliminating some junk food each week, then expanding from there. Your head and heart will thank you later.

Diabetes Prevention

A growing body of evidence suggests that our propensity towards any form of diabetes may dictate our neurodegeneration over a lifetime. The reason for this is because uncontrolled sugar levels in the bloodstream do start causing damage to the nerves, which is known as diabetic neuropathy. [18]

Experts equate Alzheimer's to type 3 diabetes because this disease is tied to the body's insulin levels, which affect the brain. Alzheimer's patients tend to have lower amounts of insulin in their brain and trouble with the insulin receptors. The deficit of insulin results in lower cognitive capabilities. After a while, this lowered state can result in permanent brain damage.

Additionally, people diagnosed with type 2 diabetes are likely to ultimately develop Alzheimer's. The reason for this is because type 2 diabetes is normally precipitated by unhealthy lifestyles, which can lead to insulin resistance or lower amounts of insulin in the body. The reason for this is because the beta cells in the pancreas that release insulin into the bloodstream after the consumption of carbohydrates can eventually become burnt out if they are overused.

The consumption of too much sugar in one's diet causes a huge release of insulin to lower the sugar levels in the bloodstream. The beta cells, however, can only secrete a certain amount of insulin during their lifetimes, and unlike other body cells, these cells can't heal themselves.

If a person develops type 2 diabetes because of an unhealthy diet, then they will struggle with lower insulin levels for the rest of their lives. This can, ultimately, cause a person's insulin levels in their brain to drop and can precipitate Alzheimer's disease.[19]

The Environment

Our daily lives and habits have more say than you may think when it comes to developing Alzheimer's. Research suggests that this evidence can boil down to something as ambient as the air we breathe. Sitting in traffic or living alongside industrial areas may seem like a nuisance at best and an environmental hazard at worst. The reality is the danger spells terror for our cognitive health, even if the damage and danger seem far off.

Air quality is one of the highest exacerbating risks of developing Alzheimer's and other forms of dementia. Studies published in 2018 found that people who were exposed to high levels of nitrogen oxide and fossil fuel combustion matter were much more likely to develop Alzheimer's. Behind that, exposure to heavy metals such as aluminum, mercury, and cadmium can also increase the risks of developing cognitive illnesses.

To minimize your risk of developing exposure to elements and factors that can increase your odds of developing

Alzheimer's, make sure you do your homework before signing any lease or deed for the property. You should feel comfortable knowing you are living in a home that is far away from pollutants in a city that has fair air quality. Get the property tested before purchasing it, and be aware of buildings that stood there before yours. If you are already in a lease or cannot get out of your current leasing situation, try limiting your time in the area as much as possible. While you may not be able to take a vacation every week, you can find a park or green space to take a stroll or read. Ask around to see if you can spend time with friends while still doing productive things you would normally do at home.

That said, it is sometimes difficult to know about all of the dangers that are lurking beneath the surface, and we do need to know where the balance is between being careful and being overly paranoid. We need to be careful of not overexposing ourselves to environmental toxins unnecessarily, but we will all be exposed to a lesser or greater degree. This is why we need to support our bodies in the best ways that we can by leading healthy lifestyles and eating foods that are high in antioxidants (which can act against some of the oxygen free radicals that affect us from the environments that we find ourselves in).

It is still important to enjoy life and the environment that you choose to live in, but it will be necessary to be careful and avoid unnecessary risks where you can.

Eating to Heal Alzheimer's

While nothing can fully stave off this terrible chronic disease, scientists have found that healthy chemicals and nutrients in some popular foods can decrease our chances of developing these diseases and increasing brain function.

As I mentioned earlier, antioxidants are greatly needed in a person's body to combat the disease-causing oxygen-free radicals that build up in a person's body because of environmental exposures. Antioxidants are chemicals that safely eliminate these toxins from a person's body and can lower the chances of developing unfortunate diseases.

Multiple different foods are filled with antioxidants, but one of the most potent antioxidants known to man is vitamin C. Vitamin C can be found in most citrus fruits and multivitamin supplements. Just increasing a person's intake of vitamin C every day can work wonders in warding off unwanted diseases.

That said, vitamin C is a very volatile vitamin and can be destroyed easily. Exposure to heat and even light can start to degrade this vitamin, which eventually makes it redundant. If you are wanting to increase your intake of vitamin C daily, then it is recommended that you consume fresh fruits to ingest the best amount of it.

On another note, vitamin C is a water-soluble vitamin and a person can't actually take too much of it. So, if you were worried about overdoing it, then you can rest assured that, that is pretty unlikely. If you do take too much, the worst that you will experience is a bit of abdominal discomfort, because vitamin C can irritate the gut in very large doses. But that symptom is harmless and fleeting.

It is advantageous to take more than you are supposed to with this vitamin because there are numerous health bene-fits from taking more than the recommended daily allowance. Most health practitioners recommend 1000 mg every day (1000% of a recommended daily allowance), but you can take more than that if you feel you need to. Some nutritionists recommend that you can take up to 1000 mg every hour to treat severe cases of illness to rapidly boost the immune system (but be warned that this amount of vitamin C may cause some intestinal discomfort).

Tea and Coffee

Caffeine has been a stimulant that has been around for several hundred years. It used to be believed that caffeine is not a healthy addition to a person's diet, but recent research has found that caffeine can have protective qualities in the brain in moderate doses.

A morning or afternoon pick-me-up can go a long way to protecting your brain from aging quicker than it should. Coffee has been suggested to slow down cognitive decline and fight against the disease. One study found evidence that drinking three to five cups of coffee daily can reduce the risk of dementia and Alzheimer's by as much as 65%. The antioxidants in coffee may help block inflammation in the brain and promote other avenues of healing.

If the caffeine giant that is "java" is that effective, then this age-defying quality rings even more true for tea, especially green tea. This simple beverage can stave off symptoms of Alzheimer's because of its catechin polyphenols, which not only come loaded with antioxidants but also fight off twists and plaques from forming.

Therefore, it is important and necessary to actually introduce caffeine into your daily diet as an adult as a precautionary measure to stave off problems with dementia later on. Do remember to keep your caffeine intake moderate, but it is healthy to include it daily. Your source of coffee and tea is very crucial as well, many coffees are laden with pesticides and fungus. Double-check your source to ensure a high-quality product.

I recommend that my patients cycle off of coffee every four weeks to avoid adrenal burnout.

Healthy Fats

If you haven't noticed yet, Omega-3 fatty acids are kind of a superfood, and they are greatly needed in your diet. Omega-3 fatty acids act as antioxidants and anti-inflammatories and help produce healthy cholesterol in the body.

Walnuts are packed with Omega-3 fatty acids, which help foster connections for over 36 neurotransmitters. These large nuts have also been shown to promote new messaging links within brain cells. Incorporating walnuts into the diet has been shown to improve cognition and memory. If you eat fish, the fattiest acid-rich catches include salmon, tuna, and herring.

If you can't consume fish products for other reasons, then oils such as coconut, flaxseed, and olive will also come in handy because they are also high in omega-3 fatty acids. Certain yogurts, soy beverages, juice, eggs, and nuts will have some form of omega-3s as well and are very easy to include in your diet.

Many people often get confused about what omega supplements to take because there are many with different variations. After all, there are also omega-6 and omega-9 fatty acids. This may seem confusing, but fortunately, research has found that omega-3 fatty acids can convert into omega-6 and omega-9 fatty acids if the body requires these acids.

It is important to note, however, that omega-6 and omega-9 fatty acids are not able to convert lower to omega-3. So, it is better to stick with omega-3 supplements or dietary inclusions because it can convert to whatever fatty acid your body requires.

Spices[20]

Including certain extra spices into your diet may seem like a strange addition, but multiple health benefits are associated with several spices. Before I discuss the healthy attributes of some spices, it is important to note that some natural substances can cause medically significant reactions with certain medications that you may be taking. I will be discussing spices that aren't known to react with other types of medications, but there are some that you may need to research before mixing them with the medications that you are currently taking.

The first spice that you should consume more of is cinnamon. Cinnamon works wonderfully in the body to lower blood sugar levels by naturally opening the channels in the cells to accept the glucose. It is important to remember that cinnamon may not be able to replace insulin, but it does significantly aid its process. The powerful, anti-diabetic effect that cinnamon has on a person's body makes it a needed addition for most people that are looking to change their lifestyles and look after their brains.

If you struggle with high blood pressure (hypertension), then it may be necessary to be on medications to lower your blood pressure. This can be aided by the consumption of hot chilies and cayenne pepper powder. The peppers work in the blood vessels and help lower the blood pressure by normalizing the volume within the vessels themselves. Chilies are known to further lower a person's blood pressure by relaxing the heart muscle so it doesn't need to contract so strongly. This double effect works very well to naturally lower a person's blood pressure.

Since you are wanting to look after your brain and preserve your memory, there are several herbs that you can introduce into your diet to improve your memory and protect your brain, but the best of the herbs is sage. Sage is a slightly strange herb because it's practically inedible when it's fresh, but has a very subtle and pleasant flavor when it's cooked or dried. Adding a few sage leaves to your roasted potatoes makes for a delicious side-dish that all of your family members will dive into.

The reason why sage directly helps combat the onset of Alzheimer's is that sage prevents the breakdown of acetylcholine in the brain. And, since Alzheimer's is precipitated by a drop in acetylcholine in the brain, then this is definitely an herb that you would want to keep including regularly.

The final two spices that will be discussed are ginger and turmeric. They have been included together because although they are different, they have powerful anti-inflammatory properties with antioxidant effects. These anti-inflammatory properties both work in the body and directly in the brain which will greatly lessen the risk of developing cognitive illnesses.

On a final note, you don't have to go out and buy supplements that have these spices in them, and you can just include them in your cooking routine. Many curries that you can make are simple and incorporate chilis, cinnamon, ginger, and turmeric so they will obviously be beneficial to you and your family… and they're delicious.

Parkinson's Disease

"Destroying everything that You've Worked for"

Much like Alzheimer's disease, Parkinson's disease is a seemingly irreversible disease that comes about slowly - eventually robbing its victims of their dignity and their ability to take care of themselves. The disorder is most likely to affect people later in life, and the likelihood of developing this disease becomes greater as the years go by – onset is correlated with increasing age. One of Parkinson's most notable characteristics is a slight tremor in the hands that progressively worsens and then begins to spread to the rest of the body.

Parkinson's is the second-most common neurodegenerative disease in modern times (behind Alzheimer's disease). More than 10 million people live with Parkinson's, and around 60,000 Americans are diagnosed with the disease annually. Both men and women are more likely to develop the disease as they get older, however, men are slightly more likely than women to develop it regardless of age. It is uncommon, but it is possible to develop Parkinson's disease at younger ages usually because of unfortunate accidental trauma to the brain, or sometimes drug abuse.[21][22]

Symptoms

People in the beginning stages of Parkinson's may find their facial expressions are limited or they may not be able to make any facial expressions at all. Speech may become soft or slurred and one's facial muscles may begin to feel unnaturally tighter. The list of potential symptoms from Parkinson's is long, and those who experience it may watch helplessly as the disease worsens.

A common misconception about Parkinson's is that many believe that it is solely related to movement. However, symptoms of Parkinson's are related to both movement and non-movement. Common symptoms include cramping, drooling, strained handwriting, dementia, memory issues, difficulty speaking, and difficulty focusing. People who suffer from Parkinson's may find themselves sweating more than normal or are excessively cold when they shouldn't be. The difficulties in the regulation of body temperature may become very irritating to people, but it is one of the earlier signs you can watch out for.

There is a myriad of different symptoms that people can experience in the beginning stages of Parkinson's and can vary according to individuals. Some may experience sleep problems with sexual dysfunction, while others may experience fatigue, weight loss, and increased dandruff. These symptoms may appear in clusters or individually. It all depends on how the disease is progressing in the individual person.

People who suffer from Parkinson's may also develop further problems in the later stages of the disease, like sleeping, vision, taste, smell, or using the restroom. Finally, people may also experience involuntary movements, pain, lost appetite, and shoulder pain is a very common occurrence.

There are several stages that people suffering from Parkinson's disease commonly experience – each stage moves on to the next as the disease progresses becoming more and more severe. The first stages are characterized by mild symptoms that normally do not interfere with daily life, including mild tremors, facial expressions, walking, and posture. In the middle stages, the patient will soon encounter walking problems, loss of balance, slowed movements, and the inability to take care of themselves.

The most advanced stage of Parkinson's includes the inability to stand or walk. People in this stage are commonly wheelchair-bound or bedridden, and they often require close, highly personalized medical care around the clock. Aside from these symptoms, someone suffering from Parkinson's may have an impaired sense of smell, difficulty sleeping, cognitive issues, fatigue, lightheadedness, sweating, constipation, and bladder symptoms.

It is a very debilitating illness and unfortunately, there is no cure (just like with Alzheimer's), but many of these symptoms are manageable with healthy diet changes, and lifestyle alterations.

Causes

Parkinson's is developed when the brain does not receive enough dopamine to carry messages to its billions of cells. As stated in chapter three, dopamine is a neurotransmitter that pertains to body movement and control. If brain cells die, the brain responds by producing less dopamine, which inhibits the brain's control over movement. The result, ultimately, is that these patients exhibit slow and strange responses and movements. Parkinson's symptoms normally begin showing when 80% of cells in the affected area of the brain have died, which is problematic because then treatment only occurs much later into the disease's progression.

Much like Alzheimer's, experts are working to determine the cause of Parkinson's. People are similarly affected by factors including genetics, environmental issues, and lifestyle choices. These can be hereditary, but often, they are seemingly formed at random. However, research has linked pesticides, altered dopamine levels within the individual, and diet, to the formation of Parkinson's. Finally, Parkinson's researchers are still looking for a cure to this day, as there is currently no recovery once someone develops the disease.

It does seem very dire and depressing, but with the right treatments, the development of Parkinson's and its symptoms can be slowed greatly. Unfortunately, when the damage is done to the brain, those areas can't be fixed because neural tissue can't generally regenerate (or if it does, it does so very slowly), but the progression can be slowed by introducing healthy nutrients and developing a healthy lifestyle to the body and, ultimately, the brain.

Genetics

Parkinson's is rarely the result of genetics, and although genetics can play a part in the development of the disease, environmental factors and exposures are much more influential. Less than 20% of Parkinson's cases can be attributed to DNA. These cases normally come up because family members hold certain genes that make them more predisposed to forming Parkinson's. [23]

Dozens of gene mutations have been linked to Parkinson's, and for reasons unknown to researchers, North African Arab Berbers and Ashkenazi Jews may be more susceptible to Parkinson's based on genetic predisposition. While we cannot control our genetics, we can mostly control the other forms of contributors to our ability to form this disease, which involves diet, exercise, and the environment. [24]

Diet and Exercise[25]

There is no singular cause for Parkinson's but rather a whole bunch of contributing factors that seem to synergize horribly together to bring pathology about. Without a single, simple cause, there can be no single simple cure; and indeed, there is no known way to cure the disease at the present state of medical knowledge.

The 'solution' to Parkinson's, as such, is to simply safeguard as best as you can from developing the disease – and that is best done by taking the best care of yourself that you possibly can to keep your heart and blood vessels healthy along with ensuring your gut health is robust and resilient. Current conventional best practice, at least in terms of functional medicine, is to make sure that you are eating from all the food groups (a varied diet) and avoid diets that tell you otherwise (like cutting out all carbs or some other unhealthy fad).

Critically important to people with brain concerns, like those with Parkinson's, is to absolutely make sure that you ingest tons of antioxidants in your diet. The best sources for the right kinds of potent anti-oxidants are usually dark fruits, a wide variety of pesticide-free organic veggies, and chocolate, the darker the better. Light-colored fruits are also great sources for antioxidants and they tend to be packed with powerful healing nutrients. The key point here is to eat a wide variety of foods, nuts, fruits, veggies, everything. The wider the variety, the better. Emphasizing food sources of nutrients, compounds, and minerals listed in part II of this book will also boost your brain's health and performance radically – basically ensuring you are doing the absolute best you could be doing to stave off not just Parkinson's disease, but any other chronic lifestyle and degenerative disorder that might be on the horizon for you. A wide variety of foods and large quantities of the right foods relative to the wrong foods will ensure a happy gut, happy heart, and happy brain – a happy healthy body and life for you.

Although particular supplements and vitamins have not been definitively linked with fighting against Parkinson's, many different factors have been investigated in the research literature into effective tools to fight AD. Most notably, vitamin C occupies much of the literature currently published, and you can bet that it is of the most potent antioxidants that a person can take for brain health whilst also being a strong candidate as a preventative supplement for Parkinson's disease too.

As a general rule of thumb, it tends to be better for you in the long run if you always try to stick to natural remedies, or natural sources of compounds to boost your health and ward off negative symptoms.

Natural compounds tend to come in tolerable concentrations and when accompanied by all the other naturally occurring things in their sources tend to have better availability and long-term results in the body. However, if things are severe, and you find yourself completely out of balance because you are suffering from a disease, then it is likely you will need to take very high concentrations of these naturally sourced compounds for a small while just to bring the body back into a semblance of balance again so that its natural systems can catch up and start doing their marvelous work for you again.

An example of a naturally occurring compound is curcumin, which is found in turmeric. Curcumin is a superstar compound for health and has many powerful effects on the body that can promote healing and optimal functioning in the right circumstances.

One drawback with curcumin is that to get therapeutic concentrations of it into the body you usually have to supplement in high doses – which can come with certain risks. However, if turmeric is increased in your diet, then day by day the cumulative effects of curcumin in your diet will have very large effects on your good health over time.

Indeed, one good way to make the curcumin in turmeric more bioavailable to the body is to also increase your black pepper intake – they work synergistically together to help the body absorb and use curcumin properly.

Another great natural compound is St. John's Wort – extracts of this plant have been shown to reduce symptoms of depression – this is a great example of a naturally sourced compound that is well tolerated with amazing benefits – in this case, to combat depression and mood slumps linked to dopamine depletion in the brain.

Natural remedies are powerful. I have already mentioned that curcumin in high doses can have powerful effects on the body. On the one hand, we want these natural compounds to have powerful effects because that is how they actually help us to heal and regain balance in our bodies. On the other hand, with that kind of power comes a certain degree of responsibility - we should take supplements carefully.

St. John's Wort, like curcumin, is another case in point. If used incorrectly it can cause problems because it can excite enzymes in the liver which can cause toxic interactions with other medications. It is always best to follow good safety guidelines when taking natural compounds for health, and also always best to do so under the supervision of an experienced healing professional.

Don't worry about this too much, in this book I have emphasized the safest options that are also the most powerful for you to use. I have also recommended those natural remedies and supplements that are readily available, affordable, and easy to use.

Eating healthily and maintaining a healthy intake of nutritious foods is just the beginning of slowing the symptoms of Parkinson's. It is also vital to maintain a regular exercise habit because it will help you regulate many of the same health factors. Fitting in about half an hour of moderate exercise four days a week is enough to help you keep your heart healthy and weight down. Regular exercise also helps you metabolize the food and other nutritious foods you are taking in.

One final note is that exercise increases the blood flow to the brain, so the brain tissue does become more oxygenated during times of exercise. Keeping your brain tissue oxygenated will slow the effects and symptoms of both Alzheimer's and Parkinson's in addition to giving your body all the other amazing benefits of exercise too. I discuss exercise in more detail later in the book.

Environmental Factors

Similar to Alzheimer's, Parkinson's can be brought on by adverse environmental conditions. There are a few different particular environmental factors that you should take special care to avoid.

Pesticides and herbicides

These have been clearly and definitively linked to incidences of early-onset Parkinson's disease. These poisons include rotenone and permethrin, which are sometimes found in mosquito-killing nets or clothes. If you know you are near a site that produces these chemicals, try to put as much physical distance from yourself and the plant as possible.

- **MPTP** is a synthetic neurotoxin that was accidentally used in the 1980s when California scientists injected synthetic heroin. The participants in the study who were intravenous drug users immediately developed Parkinson's-like symptoms. These symptoms became permanent because of the drop in dopamine in their brains.

- **Manganese exposure** may come from places where welding is predominant.
- **Organic pollutants** have been suggested to cause Parkinson's. These are most commonly known as polychlorinated biphenyls (PCBs), were used for industrial purposes. You will find these in plastics, coolants, and major electronics.
- **Solvents** in paint thinners, detergents, dry cleaning, and metal degreasing may be linked to Parkinson's.

The best way to safeguard against Parkinson's is to work towards preventing it every day. You will find that the healthier your lifestyle and the cleaner your environment, the longer you will keep your brain tissue healthy, and the longer you will be able to ward off the onset of these symptoms. Many people have to go through their entire lives without experiencing the onset of symptoms, even with genetic vulnerabilities, past exposures, and confirmed onset of the disease. Leading a healthy lifestyle can keep you healthy for decades to come.

Strong Brain Tip for Parkinson's #1:

If preventing the onset of Parkinson's to fortify your life isn't enough motivation, consider making a change for the benefit of your family and those surrounding you. Leading a healthy life will make you want to hang onto it for much longer, and there is no reason why you shouldn't do everything that you can to change the possible outcomes of developing Parkinson's.

Strong Brain Tip for Parkinson's #2:

Consult your doctor if you have noticed any change in your sense of smell. This is especially true if you cannot smell peanut butter anymore. It turns out that there is a high correlation between the loss of smell of peanut butter and Parkinson's disease. This can be a crucial early detection measure that would allow you to prevent further onset. If you do notice that there may be some underlying symptoms, don't be stubborn and avoid going to the doctor. Having the symptoms assessed by a professional can greatly slow the development of the illness if you make changes early on.

4

WHEN THINGS GO WRONG (B)
(GENERAL DEMENTIA & MIGRAINES)

Dementia: Who...? Wha...? Where...am I?

Brain tissues tend to age and deteriorate over time, but the rate at which they tend to do this is linked to a whole complex of different factors. Generally speaking, the natural degeneration of brain tissue as people age can be offset somewhat by eating healthily, exercising, and looking after our 'bio-body-suits'. In normal, healthy cases of aging, brain degeneration is measurable in terms of slight losses in memory, sharpness, and other parameters, but this slight decline over time never involves debilitating loss of function – however, in Dementia, the degeneration is so bad that there is a significant and serious loss of function that goes way beyond normal aging. People with Dementia lose major functionality in their mental performance, particularly with memory and attention, and they often ultimately experience radical changes in personality and 'sense of self' – typically Dementia patients will eventually find it difficult to manage simple day-to-day life without supervision or help of some kind.

Dementia affects some 50 million people worldwide, with 10 million new cases annually.[1] So what is dementia as compared to Alzheimer's or Parkinson's. Well, you can think of dementia as a large umbrella term that includes other kinds of disorders – a good example is Alzheimer's disease, which is a special form of dementia characterized by plaques in the brain and a very specific disease progression profile. So, dementia is a term that is used to describe a condition in a person who is having marked brain degeneration problems leading to clinically severe cognitive and psychological problems like extreme memory impairment, personality changes, and other effects. Think of dementia as meaning something close to severe biologically based confusion that massively affects day to day life.

Overall, dementias of any type tend to impair memory, comprehension (words, meaning, place, and time), language, awareness, and/or judgment. While people with dementia are fully conscious, this disease robs them of years (if not decades) of memories, hard work, social cues, or motivation to continue. Experts have statistically projected forward that the number of people suffering from dementia will likely *triple* by 2050!

The difficulty in detecting dementia is the fact that it comes on quietly and progresses very slowly. Families of loved ones with dementia often don't notice the clear decline in the affected dementia patients because they keep getting used to how that person is now, without reflecting far enough backward in time to realize the radical difference in mental performance. So, what usually happens is that people are suddenly shocked when some major problem sets in that is clearly out of the ordinary. The truth is that dementia was usually present for decades, just that at some point common sense gets violated and people only then really take notice – the realization is usually shocking, and concerning.

The most noticeable symptoms of early-stage dementia include becoming lost in familiar places, forgetfulness, and losing track of time. As the disease progresses, people with dementia will rely more on others for personal care, as they may become lost at home, forget people's names or recent events, find it hard to communicate, or change their behaviors. Late-stage dementia manifests in people completely losing awareness of time or place, difficulty walking, aggression, and difficulty recognizing friends and relatives.

Dementia occurs following gradual damage to brain cells. Thinking and behavior are affected when brain cells are unable to effectively communicate with one another. Destruction of these cells can often be a side effect of other health problems such as thyroid problems, vitamin deficiencies, excessive alcohol consumption, medication side effects, and depression.

Interestingly, temporary states of unbalanced health can mimic dementia symptoms until the state passes –in many ways people suffering from an extremely traumatic shocking event can exhibit signs of memory loss, psychological shock, and other problems. The same can be said of an extreme episode of major depression which can also affect sleep, memory, personality and motivation, mood, and behavior. But in these cases, when the depression lifts or the shock or trauma is dealt with and abates, then normal functioning returns. In the case of dementia, that functioning is lost, usually forever. Often, the transient cognitive impairment that can arise from people without dementia is linked to unbalanced neurotransmitter profiles, malnutrition, or hyper-stressful states which can be treated adequately with good nutrition, coping strategies, psychotherapy, exercise, proper sleep, or lifestyle changes as indicated.[2]

Primary Causes

As with all illnesses in the complex cerebral tissue, there can be a myriad of different factors that can ultimately cause the development of dementia. As with Alzheimer's and Parkinson's, there may be underlying genetic factors, but many of them seem to be environmentally based.

Familial links to Dementia – Understanding Your History

Having a family member who develops dementia increases your odds of eventually developing it too. Similar to Parkinson's and Alzheimer's, the risk for people whose family member has developed Alzheimer's increases by about 30%. However, most cases are not inherited from their predecessors. History of Parkinson's may also spell a history of drug abuse or indicate that one has been exposed to environmental toxins for too long.

Recent research has suggested that vitamin D deficiencies may increase people's odds of developing dementia. This study found that people who spent most of their time inside experienced a faster pace of cognitive decline. This is why people in countries in the Northern Hemisphere must consider taking vitamin D supplements to keep their levels boosted.

People that live in countries in the Southern Hemisphere rarely have vitamin D deficiencies because of the longer periods of sunlight that regularly warm these countries. Since vitamin D is one of the only vitamins that humans can produce naturally through ultraviolet ray absorption from sunlight, it is needed for people that don't want to take extra supplementation.

Understanding Dementia

There are multiple factors that one needs to understand when they are facing an illness like dementia. Many people are very scared of the potential of developing an illness that causes a cognitive decline with passing time, and many people choose to stay in denial than actually dealing with their problem.

To understand dementia, one needs to first grasp that dementia is not a single illness or problem. It is, rather, a collection of problems that ultimately cause the mental devolution of a person suffering from the illness. This collection of causes result in an illness that affects the dopamine and acetylcholine levels in one's brain and causes a miscommunication between the cells in the brain.

Researchers have been studying cognitive illnesses that affect people, but there are still many questions that haven't been answered yet, and thus far, there aren't any cures for these illnesses yet. There are medications that people can take to slow the onset of symptoms, but treating the symptom isn't the same as treating the illness.

The best way to truly treat the illness is ultimately by slowing its progression with a healthy lifestyle change. The reason why this is important is that dementia is a developing illness and will cause extreme debilitation if left untreated. People that develop dementia will ultimately struggle to take care of themselves and will require personal care and assistance practically all the time. This can put a lot of strain on relationships and can ultimately end in irreparable emotional harm to all parties involved.

Ultimately, if one does develop this type of cognitive illness, it will progress... but how quickly it progresses is all up to how the individual combats it in the beginning stages, when they first notice their symptoms. The greatest danger in the beginning stages of dementia is to ignore it and pretend like it isn't happening, because that is valuable time being lost when you could be altering your lifestyle.

Strong Brain Tip for Dementia #1:

Even small memory lapses such as forgetting your car keys, misplacing objects, or only partially completing tasks can be signs of memory issues. If you notice these symptoms are becoming common-place in your life, then don't hesitate to get them checked out by a professional.

Strong Brain Tip for Dementia #2:

Memory games can help boost areas of the brain to help increase blood flow and help remove toxic metabolites. Grab a chessboard and a partner and play a few games every week. Chess is one of the greatest games that you can play to exercise your brain. Research has found that children's IQs who play chess develop much faster than the IQs of children that don't. If chess is good enough to do that, then it will help slow the progression of dementia.

Migraines

Headaches are can hinder your quality of life greatly, and there are various reasons why they can afflict a person. Some of them range from mild to incredibly severe, and migraines fall onto the latter end of that scale.

Migraines are severe headaches that are commonly associated with pulsating or throbbing sensations, and often occur on one side of the head. The sensation may result in light and sound sensitivities, vomiting, paralysis, sweating, cold hands, inability to swallow, confusion, and nausea. For many people, migraines may be an occasional inconvenience best fixed by a day in bed and a cold compress on the eyes. But some people have migraines that don't break for days on end and are extremely debilitating.

Migraines tend to affect women more than men (because men are prone to developing cluster headaches instead, and according to men, they are worse than migraines… but this is a debatable topic), and 10% of people who suffer from them may experience attacks weekly. Less than half are treated effectively with traditional medication remedies and require either stronger medications or long periods of bed rest. In all, around one in five adults experience migraines regularly, and one in six women in the United States will experience a headache on semi-regular occasions.

Migraines are episodic, but can completely lay waste to our productivity throughout the day. When experiencing a migraine, it's best to lie still, and in a dark place so the pain will not become worse. The pain can last for as little as four hours but can last as long as three days in extreme cases. Nearly $13 billion is lost each year to the physical and emotional pain of throbbing headaches. Men on average require four days of bed rest annually and women require around six days. [3] [4]

Spot the Signs of Migraines

You may notice some physical, mental, or psychological changes in the time before the migraine sets in. This is normally the best time to start a form of treatment to prevent it from getting worse. If you are prone to migraines, and you notice that any of the following symptoms are creeping in, then it is better to take action before they set in. A natural trick to combat the migraine is placing your hands into a bath of cold water, and get into a dark room. This causes vasodilation (when your blood vessels expand or 'dilate') in the brain which may alleviate the migraine symptoms temporarily. The signs that you need to watch out for are: [5]

- Mood changes
- Loss of appetite
- Changes in digestive schedule
- Water retention
- Thirst
- Excessive urination
- Food cravings
- Exhaustion and excessive yawning
- Altered senses
- Changes in vision
- Difficulty with motor control
- Strange bouts of nausea

Unfortunately, many of these symptoms can be rather generic, but you do come to learn how your body responds according to certain stimuli. I have a friend that, personally, starts perceiving severe visual impairments before the onset of his migraines. He complains that a large black dot starts growing in the field of vision out of his right eye, and then he knows that he is going to experience the full onset of migraine within the next 20 minutes. That is quite a severe example, but he has learned to read his body and can start treating his migraines when he notices the signs.

Avoid the Triggers

As we've established in previous chapters, the fuel we put into our bodies directly affects our propensity towards migraines. Researchers over the years have asked people to modify their diets for certain foods and beverages. People who cut these items from their diets experienced fewer migraines and lost fewer days to migraines. The tests also paved the way for delivering an individualized approach to treating the illness.

Take some time to explore food's effects on your body. Over the next few weeks, consider adding in or cutting out different foods and catalog your body's responses. If you suspect that certain food items give you migraines, then avoid them.

People complain about certain food items that trigger migraines in them, and although it is not overly common, there are instances where people will experience the onset of a migraine after eating specific foods. These are normally limited to one or two food items in people that are prone to migraines, but if there are triggers like this that cause you to suffer from migraines, then it is better to avoid those food items entirely. [6]

These food items include: [7] [8] [9]

- Sodas (carbonated sugary drinks)
- Dairy products
- Processed or aged meats
- Dried fruit
- Chocolate
- Potato chips
- Nuts or seeds
- Artificial sweeteners and seasonings such as MSG (monosodium glutamate)
- Citrus fruits and bananas
- Yeast bread, grains (Gluten)
- Red wine
- Coffee or tea consumed in excess

Although there are food triggers, there are also other triggers that can cause a migraine in people, and these include: [10]

- Head trauma
- Lack of exercise
- Medication
- Artificial food additives
- Stress
- Hormonal changes

- Foods containing preservatives or large amounts of sugar
- Inflammation
- Autoimmune system issues
- Changes in sleeping patterns
- Changes in air pressure
- Bright lights or strong smells
- Environmental stressors

Use the Right Treatment

Since I am a functional medicine practitioner and prefer more naturally-based alternatives to traditional medications, I am more prone to advise more natural forms of treatments. Fortunately, there are natural remedies that are available and effective against migraines.

Petasite, or the extract from a butterbur plant, has been shown to curb migraines. This plant-based supplement is proven to reduce inflammation, especially in the walls of the heart. Around 50-75 mg of the supplement is extremely effective as a primary method of fighting migraines. When you personally look for natural remedies, search for supplements that are pyrrolizidine alkaloid-free, as taking extracts that do have these can damage the liver. [11] General side effects of this supplement include drowsiness, fatigue, burping, headaches (which can be problematic when you're taking it to treat a migraine, but fortunately, this is not a common side-effect), asthma, diarrhea, pruritus, upset stomach, and itchy eyes. [12]

Petasites may cause allergic reactions in those who are allergic to marigolds, daisies, chrysanthemums, and ragweed. Do exercise caution when using these remedies, because some people are still allergic to other plants that are similar to the remedy that they are taking, and allergic responses can occur. Always consult your health care provider before beginning a new supplement. [13]

Magnesium can be taken in much larger quantities than Petasites. At least 300 mg of the mineral daily can help relieve migraines. The mineral can help optimize serotonin levels and aid in bolstering blood cells. Taking magnesium by mouth can result in diarrhea, nausea, vomiting, and gastrointestinal problems. This is due to the relaxation of muscle tissue that occurs with magnesium. Make sure to reduce the dosage to eliminate these side effects. [14] [15]

Other natural remedies that you can look into are riboflavin supplements, coenzyme Q10 tablets, omega-3 gel tablets, and phytofluene. These natural remedies aren't great at treating a migraine immediately, but long-term usage of these supplements will greatly reduce the frequency and overall severity of any future migraines. [16] [17]

Strong Brain Tip for Migraines #1:

Journaling is the simplest way to listen to your body. Record every instance of migraines. Having a working catalog of every instance your migraines flare-up will make it easier to identify triggers and make changes accordingly.

Strong Brain Tip for Migraines #2:

If you experience a migraine, try dipping your hands in cold water for as long as your hands can take the temperature. This is an easy way to mitigate the factors that worsen migraines.

A Personal Recommendation from a Patient Who used to suffer from Migraines

I have employed alternative medicine techniques while treating patients over the years, and although they may take longer to work than traditional medications, they are still more effective in the long-run because of the overall benefits of employing these natural techniques and using natural remedies.

This is a direct quote from one of the patients that I helped during my career:

"Thanks to Dr. Strong, I am now headache free and able to be the mother my daughter deserves, and I desire to be. I would recommend Dr. Strong to any and everyone. He will not only spend the time needed to get you feeling better — but functioning better for everyday life."

— GRACE S.

EXPOSURE!

Your Everyday Environment Impacts Your Brain

Do you ever feel different after visiting someplace entirely new or eating something that does not agree with your stomach? Whatever new thing you just experienced or new snack that you sampled, do you really know what's in the air, what was in the product? While it's theoretically great for us to experience new things and expand our horizons, our bodies are creatures of habit and struggle with change.

You may be able to find the cause of your allergies in your diet or responses to chemicals in different surroundings. For instance, if you did not grow up drinking cow's milk, you may find that drinking milk or eating dairy products as an adult, upsets your gut health. This is because your body is not used to ingesting this nutrient in that form. However, many of our problems can be traced back to the things we experience that are not so apparent. For better or worse, we absorb a lot from the environments in which we were raised.

It's normal for our bodies to make assumptions and corrections based on the messages we've received from the world. While you may be fully aware that something is not going to harm you, your body does not understand the context or nuances that make us open to trying new things. But this can have varying degrees of influence on our mental health, ranging from bothersome to borderline deadly.

Forms of Exposure

There are two types of exposure that you will need to keep in mind when you are thinking about the types of influential factors that have influenced you over your lifetime:

1. **Acute exposure.** Hours or days after we expose ourselves to a toxic environment or substance, we may feel the symptoms of the exposure. After removing ourselves from this location or removing the substance from our lives, we may have the feeling subside.

2. **Chronic exposure** is much more serious. This form of exposure can materialize over the years, or even decades. Along the way, the exposure will inhibit or disturb our cell functions. Over time, and in more severe cases, chronic exposure can lead to neurodegenerative diseases like Alzheimer's disease and Parkinson's disease.

Everyday Items that Could Pose Risk

There might be a few items lying around your home and garage that have the potential to impair your cognitive capabilities. It may seem like a strange thing to say that the materials you use to clean your home can actually be harming you, but several common household cleaning chemicals do cause more harm than good.

- **Detergents and cleaners.** These products that may keep your dishes, clothes, and surfaces clean may be costing you some mental clarity. Laundry detergents may contain cationic, non-ionic, or anionic enzymes that, if ingested, can cause vomiting, convulsions, shock, and induce comas. Keep a lookout for non-ionic detergents—they may irritate your eyes or skin, and prolonged exposure to detergent may cause asthma. When it comes to all-purpose cleaners, sodium hypochlorite and ammonia can cause irritation in the eyes, nose, skin, or throat.

- **Bleach liquid and vapors** can cause nausea, vomiting, stomach irritation, esophageal damage, and dermatitis. When mixed with ammonia, bleach can release poisonous gas and hurt your ability to breathe.

- **Oven cleaners** are dangerous to breathe in or touch because they usually contain lye, an extremely corrosive chemical that can burn you. Look for non-toxic oven cleaners that do not contain lye to be safe.

- **Antibacterial cleaners** usually contain some sort of pesticide to eradicate germs. Wear latex gloves if you are cleaning with antibacterial cleaner and avoid making contact with your skin or eyes.

- **Window cleaner** also contains ammonia and isopropanol. If inhaled or ingested, they can result in death, unconsciousness, or drowsiness.

- **Air fresheners** may make everything smell better, but they contain a few different chemicals n cause cancer and brain damage, including lehyde, p-dichlorobenzene, aerosol nts, and petroleum distillates. Instead of using air fresheners, consider using baking soda to neutralize foul odors.

- **Carpet cleaners** are one of the most common sources of health issues that disappear after a couple of days. The fumes that come from the cleaners and the ammonium hydroxide, naphthalene, and perchloroethylene can cause disorientation, sleepiness, nausea, loss of appetite, and dizziness.

- **Mothballs** may seem like an inconvenience at worst, however, naphthalene and p-dichlorobenzene are both hazardous chemicals that can spell danger for you. In the short term, mothballs may cause dizziness or headaches and possibly inflame your throat or eyes. If left unchecked, they may result in your forming cataracts and sustaining liver damage.

- **Antifreeze** may not come across your radar unless you have a car you drive and get checked. However, the chemical is toxic if inhaled and can cause dizziness.

- **Paint** can be a common default for people looking for the high of a legal drug. However, latex paint can give you a headache and irritate your nose, eyes, and throat if it contains formaldehyde. Oil-based paint can result in dizziness, fatigue, headaches, and nausea if inhaled. In the long term, paint can cause air circulation problems and lead to issues in the blood.

Mold

Have you come into contact with damp places lately or been in buildings that lacked overall maintenance care? Drywall and sheetrock are two materials that have become more commonplace in recent years for being cheap and are known for developing mold. When coupled with moisture, no ventilation, and the right external conditions, mold can create problems in the brain and body in the days and weeks to come.

Full disclosure: mold itself doesn't inherently harm us. At almost any point in time, you are inhaling some sort of mold. Mold growth is a natural part of life and is not something all should fear. However, if we ever become sick from mold, it is most likely because our bodies have become inundated with mold and our immune system is attacking our body in the process.

There are two different ways in which you may be affected by mold growth: mold toxicity and mold allergies. Mold allergies primarily cause a slight fever with little to no other distinguishable symptoms. As it may sound, mold toxicity is much more dangerous.

The symptoms of mold toxicity are often misdiagnosed as manifestations of other diseases like irritable bowel syndrome, fibromyalgia, multiple sclerosis, and a leaky gut – especially in people who are overly sensitive to the presence of molds in their bodies. In many such cases, the inflammatory immune responses to mold toxins seen in sensitive people can make it very difficult to accurately diagnose and treat the actual cause of the issue.

The symptoms from toxic mold exposure may not always be apparent. In many cases, these symptoms are ones that creep slowly into our daily lives before taking our quality of life hostage. Symptoms include depression, attention issues, insomnia, brain fog, and anxiety. Not everyone is susceptible to the negative symptoms from mold growth but those that are suffering the most.

You may have felt crazy if you experienced these issues without knowing the cause; I assure you that is not the case. You owe it to yourself to consult with a physician or professional to run tests in the places you visit the most frequently, then consider whether a change is in order. A simple test you can perform is

To combat the malignant effects of mold, Vitamin D has been theorized as a boosting agent against mold and is good for fighting the effects of mold growth.

Heavy Metals

Heavy metals can wreak havoc on the nervous system. We need to know this fact, and how it is we are often exposed to levels far beyond what would be the case in a natural setting.

- **Manganese** is one of the first heavy metals that one needs to be aware of because overexposure to manganese can result in a loss of libido, delayed response time, memory recall issues, loss of coordination, and hallucinations. In its worst form, those that have a form of manganese poisoning experience symptoms similar to Parkinson's disease. These symptoms in these patients can also become permanent if the exposure occurs for long enough. The danger of taking in too much manganese is mostly due to airborne issues.
- **Iron deficiencies** in children can permanently stunt their learning capabilities. However, too much iron can put you at risk for a plethora of heart problems, bone density issues, and liver disease. At its worst, too much iron can speed up the progression of Alzheimer's disease and Parkinson's disease, among other diseases. Overload can happen due to multiple factors, whether it stems from genetics, too many vitamin supplements, and/or underlying health issues.

- **Cadmium poisoning** can bring out more general symptoms, which include fever, trouble breathing, and muscle problems. It is most often found in industrial workspaces.
- **Copper deficiency** has a small book's worth of deficiencies listed alongside it, ranging from emotional outbursts, skin sensitivities, poor immune function, and lowered dopamine generation. Chronic pain and joint pain are two of many horrible symptoms. Too much copper, on the other hand, and in an already stressful situation can lead to over stimulations as well as anxiety and depression.

These heavy metals are only to name a few, and there are many more that need to be taken into consideration according to the different types of environments that you may find yourself in. We do need to consume many of these minerals in micro-quantities for healthy homeostasis in our bodies, but we do need to keep in mind that too much of those minerals can become very dangerous.

Chemical Toxins

Adjuvants in vaccines are supposed to boost our immune systems. It is no doubt that vaccines are crucial in modern medicine for safeguarding ourselves and loved-ones from diseases we would have thought were incurable merely decades ago. However, I have found one preservative, aluminum hydroxide, that can cause issues to occur whenever we do our part to inoculate ourselves against these diseases. Some of the hidden chemicals in vaccines can linger in our systems longer than expected and can cause cognitive issues and chronic fatigue.

At the risk of sounding like an elementary school "scared straight" program, a simple habit may be hurting your brain function: smoking. It is a common, yet detrimental habit. Lighting up a cigar or cigarette is calming for some, and science backs this up; within every tobacco product you smoke resides nicotine, a chemical that imitates the job that neurotransmitters are supposed to do. Nicotine mimics the feel-good sensation that dopamine produces. As time goes on, you build a tolerance to nicotine and require more to generate that same sensation. Addiction is the worst short-term side effect. In the long-term, smokers experience cognitive decline faster than their non-smoking counterparts. If that wasn't bad enough, smokers have been suggested to have a higher chance of developing dementia.

Secondhand smoke, as it is dangerous to smokers, is just as dangerous for people around smokers. In addition to putting people at risk for a plethora of cardiovascular diseases and trouble breathing, smokers are also inadvertently setting people up for decreased brain function. Smoking causes the blood vessels in your body to become fragile leading to decreased blood flow. With decreased blood flow to the brain, there is a greater chance of developing cognitive issues.

You may know the chemical glyphosate as the chemical in Roundup that kills weeds. The World Health Organization ruled in 2015 that the chemical is probably carcinogenic. Some experts fear that using Roundup over the long term will create a recipe for cognitive decline and other brain issues. Glyphosate is most commonly seen in the Midwest United States where farming is a way of life. However, this is also contained in GMO (genetically modified organisms) foods we consume today such as corn and soy products.

Bisphenol A is a common chemical used to harden plastic and it is often found on items like compact discs, water bottles, and canned items. Experts have determined that even when exposed to this chemical in modest amounts, it could stunt memory and learning as well as develop depression. Be wary of where your containers are coming from and avoid items that have long been exposed to extreme temperatures.

Environmental stressors also play a huge part in the types of dangers that we are exposed to daily. Not all of the dangers, real or perceived, might be chemicals. The nurturing you

receive from your home, pets, and loved ones indicate much about what your brain chemistry might look like if these stresses are commonplace. Examples of stress can be feeling fundamentally unsafe at home, whether that is due to your neighborhood or the people or person you are sharing a home with. Perhaps there is a conflict going on with your family. If there is no familial strife, there is always the possibility of financial well-being coming into play. If you are a parent or are in charge of anything else that holds life, you may be grappling with how or whether you can afford to pay for another living being and yourself to eat through the end of the month. Whatever the reason, emotional distress can be detrimental to your brain-gut axis by upsetting your stomach. Emotional stress can materialize as anxiety, depression, loss of appetite, irritability, and lack of sleep.

Some forms of emotional stress are difficult to escape. We may be stuck in abusive spousal relationships or maybe the product of abuse from our parents. Nevertheless, it is important to seek out a medical opinion to detect possible stressors in your environment and make a change for you and your brain's sake. Perhaps a mantra for this book should be, "It's never too late," because it is not too late to reclaim your life from the stress within and around you. If you are in an abusive relationship, reach out for help in a way that does not endanger you or your loved ones.

Multiple environmental factors can exacerbate the onset of certain cognitive diseases, and although we may not be able to avoid them entirely, we may be able to reduce the effects of these stressors. Daily exercising and healthy lifestyle choices help our bodies cope with the constant environmental toxins and stressors that we are exposed to, and can help reduce the chances of these types of diseases.

Although studies still must be done to form a consensus of its origins, Parkinson's disease has been linked to factors including diet, exposure to metals, well water consumption, pesticides, and rural living. All of these can increase the odds of developing Parkinson's.[1]

Strong Brain Tip for Exposure #1:

Cognitive issues due to environmental toxins can be tough to resolve. Consult with a seasoned physician to address these issues properly. If you notice that you are experiencing strange or unusual symptoms (no matter how small), it may be better to have them checked out. Some of these diseases may not be curable, but they are very manageable if diagnosed early on.

Strong Brain Tip for Exposure #2:

Exposure to toxins at work, home, or out and about is common and actually inevitable. But it is prudent to keep track of the places that you go to, so if something does happen, you can trace the "exposure" back to where it occurred and possibly find the causing agent. If you can, take a vacation, move, work from home, or stay in a different location and make note of any changes.

II

TOOLS FOR OPTIMAL BRAIN HEALTH

|SUPPLEMENTS | LIFESTYLE STRATEGIES |
EATING RIGHT

6

HAPPY GUT, HAPPY BRAIN, HAPPY YOU!

Gut Health and the Microbiome Affects ALL Health

The gut microbiome is comprised of many different variations of tiny (micro) organisms including bacteria, viruses, and some others. Some estimates of the total number of organisms in the microbiome ranges between 30 and 50 trillion.[1] 30 trillion is a mind-bogglingly huge number. To put this number in perspective, the estimated number of members in our microbiome is about as many as the total number of human cells in the entire human body (estimated at roughly 37 trillion).[2] Really sit and think about this fact... if you start to feel a little uncomfortable, then that is probably a sign that you are coming to realize that when we consider ourselves to be a human body, then we are also identifying ourselves as a half-human, half bacterial colony – a staggering thought.[3]

Bacteria are not the most numerous members of our microbiome, viruses are.[4] [5] For the most part, people think of viruses and bacteria as enemies of health. While this is true in the case of unbalanced colonies of viruses and bacteria that infect us and cause damage to the body, this is not true generally. There are many helpful viruses and bacteria and these helpful viruses and bacteria are what we refer to when we refer to the microbiome. The viruses of our microbiome can be located inside the bacteria that make their home there and largely their activity is most strongly felt in the gastrointestinal system (GIT).

What roles do these apparently helpful viruses have? They help to repair the genetic material of the helpful bacteria in the gut. These viruses also allow bacteria to alter their gene sequences to adapt to the ever-changing environment of the GIT. The combined activity of these trillions of tiny organisms and viruses helps us to do several important things critical to the health of the body. Effectively the relationship is mutually beneficial and wholly friendly and positive. The microbiota benefit by having a comfortable place to live, and the human body benefits by being 'gifted' many different abilities.[6] The benefits the symbiotic association of the microbiome and the human body are so numerous that some researchers consider the microbiome to be a sort of 'organ' in its own right.[7]

Briefly, the benefits and abilities that the microbiome organ(ism) confers on the human body are listed below:

- Affects the rate of maturation of the body.
- Confers digestive advantage:[8]
- Enables the digestion of plant sugars (plant polysaccharides)
- Enables the absorption and generation of many important vitamins and lipids that would otherwise be completely unavailable to our bodies. Examples include vitamin K, most B-vitamins, and certain lipids to name a few classes of molecule.[9]
- Directly affects the level of our basic metabolism and is therefore important for gaining and losing weight as well as accounting for energy expenditure and production.[10]
- A healthy microbiome improves the nutritional value of the food we eat because it allows the proper, complete, and efficient extraction of almost every available nutrient. This is so because key enzymes and metabolic processes within bacteria in the microbiome serve to break down foods and liquids in ways that our bodies cannot – A little bit

like having an outsourced biological mechanism of health.[11]

- Our GIT can produce and receive neurochemical signals because it can produce neuroendocrine signaling molecules as well as having its own receptor sites. In a sense our "gut feeling" is a scientific reality, we almost do have a second brain, although at a seemingly more primordial level. This relationship between the brain and the GIT is referred to as, "the gut-brain axis" in the research literature. Although research into this axis is still in its relatively early days, what is known at present is that our GIT and its functioning directly affect mood, behavior, and cognitive functioning because of the production of neurotransmitters and their receptor sites. Very importantly the gut-brain axis is heavily involved in regulating the body's stress response in addition to memory, mood, and attention.[12] [13]

- Finally, the microbiome is a key player in our immunity. It is thought to be a central player in how the immune system develops as well as how it functions and responds to the demands of the internal and external environment.[14] [15] [16] [17]

The GIT microbiome is extremely important for your health with relevant effects on digestion, nutrition, stress and anxiety, moods, attention, and intelligence. Look after your internal zoo and they will look after you. Realize that whenever you eat or drink, whatever you put into your gut is not just for YOU but also for 30 Trillion other 'people' – if they are 'happy' YOU are happy, if they work properly then YOU work, think, feel and digest properly.

How Your Microbiome Develops from Young

Research seems to indicate that our microbiome develops from birth via exposure to bacteria and viruses. Our first exposure is to the internal environment of the mother, first in utero, then in the vagina. The next contact point can be the skin of the mother, doctor, or midwife - after this initial exposure, our microbiome grows and changes according to the vagaries of chance encounters between the individual and the environment. It has been noted that normal healthy human immune system development and maturation is linked to the changes and development of the microbiome and vice versa, they are correlated.[18] [19]

Research has documented the initial bacterial composition of the microbiome and its subsequent changes. Initially, it is the place of birth[20] and style of birth[21] that are both factors in the specific bacterial colony compositions of the early microbiome. Vaginally born babies usually have Lactobacillus bacterial colonies, whilst caesarian babies tend to have staphylococcus, corynebacterium, and propionibacterium colonies – the last three are typically found on the skin and other surfaces of the environment. Finally, home births versus hospital births are also linked to differing microbiome compositions.[22] [23]

The initial diversity of the microbiome usually stabilizes at around 100 different species of bacteria, however by the age of three years (roughly) the diversity increases by approximately one order of magnitude (10 times as many) and at this stage of diversity, the microbiome resembles that of an adult human's microbiome. Minor or slight variances in the composition of the microbiome are observed at varying times during normal human development (e.g. puberty and menopause) but the truth is that at any one time in our lives the microbiome changes in composition to reflect the multi-factorial demands of the external and internal environment of the body. The gut microbiome should be viewed as a sort of living entity in the sense that it is never static and unchanging, it changes with the times and seamlessly reflects the particular factors of any current circumstance – what we are eating, drinking, our emotions, everything.[24]

For completeness and interest's sake, a list of the typical bacterium usually found in the microbiome follows:

- Bifidobacterium
- Lactobacillus
- Bacteroides
- Clostridium
- Escherichia
- Streptococcus
- Ruminococcus

In healthy individuals, no particular species of bacteria will radically dominate the microbiome population over any other. It can happen that in response to our habitual patterns of behavior and dietary choices that some bacteria will begin to predominate. In some of these cases, if the unbalanced GIT microbiome is particularly inefficient or harmful then pathological symptoms may occur – such as nutrient deficiencies, energy shortages, and other symptoms. So, those factors that promote a healthy balanced gut environment tend to support the functioning of all needed gut microorganisms in appropriate ratios. Generally speaking, appropriate exercise, sufficient water intake, good dietary fiber intake, and a varied and interesting diet all tend to help keep a lively happy gut microbiome.[25]

On the other hand, if we consume antibiotics, too much sugar, too little water, or are constantly under stress then we are likely to have an unbalanced or deficient gut microbiome.[26] Taking antibiotics is particularly lethal for our micro-organismic helpers. When we take antibiotics we effectively declare chemical and biological warfare on all the bacteria in the body. To borrow a horrifying phrase from the American War Machine's foreign policy, our antibiotic military activities come with 'unfortunate collateral damage'.

To combat the effects of antibiotics we can take what are called probiotics. Probiotics are specially prepared helpful and friendly bacteria that are taken following a course of antibiotics to repatriate and recolonize the gut with helpful bacteria. This is helpful, but, one can take probiotics to rebalance an unbalanced gut microbiome even when we haven't taken antibiotics. This can be especially helpful when we change our long-standing habitual activities to support total all-round health. Changing our diet and exercise patterns recalibrates our microbiome and supplementing with probiotics when we do this can help the microbiome reach a good state quickly with great beneficial diversity.

What You Eat Determines How You Think & Feel

What if I told you the things you put into your body directly impact your mood? This may seem like a bit of an unusual statement dent... but what if those foods that boost your mood weren't the cookies, chips, or sweets you'd normally reach for?

So, it turns out to be more complicated than that. The food you put into your body affects an entire ecosystem of microscopic bacteria that live in your stomach and intestines. You would believe that no bacteria is the ideal situation... However, the billions upon billions of bacteria living inside you help balance everything from your mood to your immune system.

There are good and bad bacteria that can influence us. It is important to know and remember that the bacteria within your gut are very beneficial to the overall homeostasis (balance) in your body. These bacteria control everything from the absorption of certain nutrients to directly affecting bowel movements.

A notable example of this is when a person takes certain medications that are directly influenced by the bacteria in a person's gut. Birth control pills are directly influenced by the bacteria in the gut and are not properly absorbed if the bacterial concentration is lower than normal. The estrogen and progesterone balance from the pills are absorbed by the gut bacteria and transferred through the intestinal lining and into the bloodstream. If any medications are taken that can affect the gut bacteria (like antibiotics and certain antihistamines) then a woman can fall pregnant during this time if she isn't careful with her partner, because she wouldn't be absorbing the correct balance of hormones to prevent pregnancy.

Studies suggest that our gut can hold up to a thousand different forms of bacteria. When everything exists in harmony, the stomach operates well, and in turn, so does the brain. At many points, when we get sick, it is our body's bacteria that have been thrown out of whack for some reason or another.

Our brain is tuned in to everything that goes right or wrong in these bacteria, but the gut is also tuned into the brain. Experts have suggested that 90% of serotonin receptors are located in the gut, and, therefore, can directly influence a person's mood. Sometimes, when people are prescribed anti-depressants, they may experience side effects including diar-rhea, gastrointestinal problems, or nausea because of the types of effects that these drugs have on the bacterial balance in the gut.

The gut tells the central nervous system when things are going wrong, and sends certain signals accordingly. Some of these signals are a result of what our micro-biomes learned when we were young and respond accordingly to specific stimuli. Other factors that influ-ence our microbiomes and microflora can be environ-mental stressors according to how stressed we are. Finally, we need to be cognizant of the fact that some factors influence our gut bacteria that are predetermined in the womb.

We spend our time in the womb eating off the nutrients and energy our mothers take in. After that, we are on our own. The result is a stomach that ages and breaks down much faster than we age as humans.

A distressed gut occurs when bacteria and other chemicals permeate the lining in our stomach. We can keep our all-encompassing system of bacteria in our stomachs due to a protective lining that shields us from the "bad stuff." The barrier protects the inside from the effects of the outside world as well and protects us when things go wrong.

The intestines require a lot of communication to function adequately—after all, the GI tract is more than 30 feet in most adults. The areas between cells are a major line of defense in protecting the stomach and the outside world. We rely on proteins from our diets to facilitate these tight connections between cells in the wall.

When this barrier is broken, we may ultimately suffer from what is known as leaky gut syndrome. This syndrome occurs when there is a break in the continuum of tissue in the intestinal walls, which then allows bacteria and other harmful toxins to pass through the mucosal membranes of the intestinal walls and into a person's bloodstream.[27]

This disease process is, unfortunately, very difficult to diagnose, but it does contribute to a myriad of other health problems. Continuous barrier-breaking will lead to neurodegenerative diseases and muddle communication between the central nervous system and the gut. In turn, the gut will not operate properly and will reduce the capacity to absorb B-vitamins and other nutrients.

Just as the gut and the brain are complicated in their own right, so are the connections between them. The two create a network of feelers and receptors that include:

- **Intestinal microbiota:**
- There is a strange connection between the bacteria in the gut and the overall balance in the body. These microbiota and microflora send signals to the brain (and receive signals in return) that influence the interplay of brain balance and gut movement. It can influence the immune system, digestive system, and metabolic support, and it can prevent colonization by pathogens. Changes in microbiota are all it takes to bring on a leaky gut and other intestinal problems.[28] This will then influence immune activation, then cytokine production before causing the blood-brain-barrier to break down. Cytokines are messengers the immune system uses to communicate within itself and with

other parts of the body, using the central nervous system as a vehicle.

- **The central nervous system:**
- This is one system that is influenced by several factors and developed early in life. The stress that we experience early in life has been suggested to influence stress response later in life, and thus, how the gut-brain axis is shaped. Microbiota are connected to the central nervous system and can lead to hepatic encephalopathy, which can lead the way to tremors, dementia, stunted cognition, and comas.

Other systems include:

- The neuroendocrine system
- (A system of nerves and glands that keep the body balanced)
- The parasympathetic system
- (The part of the nervous system that automatically calms things down)
- The sympathetic nervous system
- (The part of the nervous system that automatically 'wakes and readies for action')
- The enteric nervous system (The nervous system that links to your Gut)

- The neuro-immune system (The part of the immune system that looks after the nerves)

Many of these examples that are included may seem foreign, but that is not a problem. You are not reading this book to become a doctor, but you are reading it to understand yourself, your body, and your brain a little more clearly. It can be clearly seen that several different aspects are influenced by the connection between the central nervous system and a person's GI tract. This is why it is imperative to keep the gut healthy to maintain these different relationships with the central nervous system and keep them all healthy.

There's a growing body of research that suggests that the gut and the brain are linked. When we become involved in head injuries and brain traumas, such as concussions, our guts will inevitably suffer as a consequence. As a result, lingering issues in the gut prolong neurological issues and vice versa. Our overall health is driven directly by how we fuel our bodies, the falls we take, and the environments we live in.

The choices we make during meals and the snacks in-between can go a long way in defining our health. The food we digest fosters bacterial growth and healthy development in our stomachs and intestines. Our gut is full of a myriad of different types of bacteria, so having these in the stomach and intestines is needed and a good thing. As you'll see later in the book, too much or too little of certain bacteria can be bad for your health.

Ever heard of the phrase, "You are what you eat"? As trite as it may sound, they were truly onto something. I mentioned briefly how the antioxidants, fatty acids, and minerals in whole foods helps our brains, and thus, our whole bodies, function. It seems easy, right?

Much like recent technological advancements and trends have made prioritizing our brain functions complicated, the proliferation of unhealthy habits has made keeping a healthy diet more difficult. For obvious proof, look around at what is most readily available. Fast food and pre-prepared meals in grocery stores are laden with low-nutrient, but high-calorie food items.

It appears that healthy items are more expensive. Consequently, especially in low-income neighborhoods, fresh, plant-based foods are unavailable. Our culture's obsession with unhealthy fats and sugar-laden, simple carbohydrates has garnered a notorious classification among medical experts as the Western diet, which adds inches to our waistline and years to our brain's age. It is easy to eat unhealthily, but we are cutting our lives short because of it.

The Western Diet & the Gut-Brain-Axis (GBA)

The western diet is one that is laden in the foods that are easiest to reach in the western world. Sugary beverages, salty snacks, and simple, unhealthy foods are cheap and convenient for both those looking to make a profit and those looking for a quick and seemingly filling meal. However, consuming these foods can negatively impair our ability to take in and process information. Diets, especially ones high in sugar and sweetening additives like HFCS (high fructose corn sugar), may create too many bad bacteria in the brain, as do excess intakes of fat and sugar. Of course, many of these foods have been made to be extra tasty and extra desirable.

It is important to remember that many of these food items may seem appealing at first. They are made sweeter or richer by adding in unhealthy additives. But, these types of inclusions will make the gut more toxic because the good bacteria will not thrive in the unhealthy environments that processed foods produce. The Brain-Gut axis is definitely far too toxic in the majority of people that follow an unhealthy western diet.[29]

The Link between an Unhealthy Gut and Depression[30]

Mental health disorders can be traced to feelings of emotional inflammation and stress, as well as fatigue and altered moods. Other things that are linked to emotional inflammation include diabetes, obesity, insulin resistance, and high cholesterol. An unhealthy body and an unhealthy gut will have a direct link to a person's overall outlook on life. People that struggle with unhealthily low bacterial levels in their guts do tend to struggle with more depressed states of mind than those that stick to healthier eating plans.

Maintaining a healthy gut can help reduce the effects of emotional inflammation, mental outlook, and overall brain power. Many factors can lead to altered senses of self-worth and depression, but people that constantly fuel themselves with unhealthy foods will inevitably start feeling more depressed than they should.

Several different types of nutrients and vitamins processed foods lack. Some of these examples include: folate, iron, omega-3 fatty acids, selenium, thiamine, magnesium, potassium, vitamin B12, vitamin B6, zinc, and vitamin C. There are obviously many other nutrients and vitamins that are low in processed foods, but these make up the majority of them. This is why you see labels on processed foods that state that they have been fortified with vitamins and minerals.

Many people actually think that they will be able to find a way around this, by taking supplements to compensate for their unhealthy diets, but this does not work in the way that many people expect. Although taking supplements is recommended, supplements can't help your body compensate for the high amount of saturated fats, salt, low fiber contents, and refined sugars that are hidden in fast foods. It is important to remember that supplements are important, but they can't replace a healthy diet.

Everyone's food sensitivities differ. However, a common thread has emerged among people who suffer from poor gut health:

- **Gluten** seems to irritate far more people than it did in the past and is one of the most common "food allergies" that occurs today. That said, many people aren't actually allergic to gluten, but have a serious imbalance of their gut bacteria, which upsets their digestive processes. Many people who believe that they are allergic to gluten are actually just experiencing upset gut-balances from poor diets. And, when they changed their diets and included healthier substitutions, then their guts were much more "content."

- **Too Many Calories:** We are beholden to the western diet, which is one filled with processed foods, fats, refined sugars, and carbohydrates. The diet as a whole stimulates the production of two types of bacteria into overdrive, which promotes obesity and inflammation in the gut. Consuming too many calories in one's diet will obviously influence an individual's weight gain, but a person needs to remember that they should still consume the correct amount of calories daily.

Healthy foods do still have a certain amount of calories, which need to be taken into consideration when consuming food daily. Speaking generally, and depending on your particular activity levels and other factors like pregnancy, illness, and so on, women should still consume roughly 2000 calories per day, while men should consume roughly 2500 calories per day on average because of their increased muscle masses. Less than these amounts could result in a person's body starting going into 'starvation mode' which will release cortisol to convert extra calories into body fat.

Although people may consume fewer calories in a daily period, they may still put on weight. After all, their bodies are trying to store energy reserves because they are starving themselves. It is important to remember that consuming too many calories will make one put on weight, but consuming too few calories will not produce the desired results. Anyone that is trying to get healthy must consume the correct amount of healthy calories every day to ensure that their metabolism stays boosted. (Check the following resource to see how many calories you would need a day depending on your particular circumstances. https://tdeecalculator.net/)

- **Dairy,** like gluten, also seems to have acquired a bad reputation over the past couple of decades because of the food allergies that people seem to experience because of it. There is a lot of debate surrounding how severe some of these allergies are, but there are many calories that can be cut out when choosing the right types of dairy products.

Far too many people consume dairy products that are openly high in fats. Any dairy products that state that they are high in fat or cream should actually be avoided for the most part. The reason for this is because those unnecessary creamy additions are laden with unnecessary calories and cause a person to consume too many calories in one sitting and actually irritate the gut. Low-fat options are just as tasty as full-fat products and do not cause a person to consume too many calories without realizing it.

There is another added benefit of consuming low-fat dairy products in the form of yogurts. Yogurts are naturally high in the same "good" bacteria that one needs in their stomach and intestines. Eating yogurts that are lower in calories will be a great addition to one's daily dietary intake and will also aid in keeping one's gut bacteria levels high.

- **Refined sugar:** Refined sugar has the possibility of damaging a person's liver when consumed excessively. Additionally, cutting down on refined sugars has been shown to help with breathing and, in turn, combat depression. Some studies have shown that refined sugar can increase insulin resistance and metabolic syndrome, so they do need to be consumed sparingly. Refined sugar has been shown to alter people's breathing after consuming large amounts.

Understanding what to consume is a vital part of living a healthy lifestyle. Many people believe that they need to cut sugar out completely of their diets, but this is not the case. Carbohydrates are divided into complex and simple categories, and both are important to function healthily.

Complex carbohydrates are the starches that people would consume daily. This means that any grains and bread products that are consumed will, inevitably, be converted into sugars during their digestive processes. Simple carbohydrates are any forms of sugars that are consumed and become instantly accessible in a person's bloodstream as an energy source.

People need to consume carbohydrates to adequately fuel their bodies during daily periods, but the right types of carbohydrates are needed for this task. It is better to consume carbohydrates that are less refined than others (sweet potato or starches with high fiber contents) because it will allow for a slower absorption of energy during the digestive period.

- **Alcohol** is a highly-debated topic when it comes to a person's health. Alcohol can be very detrimental to a person's well-being and can result in liver and other organ damage if abused. That said, there are some health benefits to alcohol that need to be mentioned.

Some alcohols are very high in calories and will make people put on weight if they are drunk in excess. Beers and cocktails are two examples of alcoholic beverages that need to be avoided. Beer has a high carbohydrate value because of the grains and yeast needed to brew the beer, and cocktails are generally quite high in excess sugar. This means that these beverages can cause unnecessary weight gain if consumed unnecessarily.

Other alcoholic beverages can be considered if you want to stay healthy but still consume something on a special occasion. Red wine and other stronger spirits, like whiskey, do still have calories, but they do have other antioxidants that are beneficial to one's body when taken in moderation.

Alcohol doesn't have to be excluded entirely from one's diet, but it does need to be taken carefully and on the odd occasion, instead of an every-day regularity. As you will come to find out, many food substances can still be enjoyed in moderation without causing irreparable harm.

- **Foods with low nutritional value but high-fat content** are becoming more and more prevalent with the ever-increasing availability of fast-food outlets. These types of foods are saturated with unhealthy fats and refined sugars. They quintessentially have very little nutritional value for the number of calories that they pack into your system when you consume them.

The consumption of these types of foods do interfere with a person's gut bacteria and will ultimately cause havoc to a person's digestive processes when consumed in excess.

It is better to greatly limit your intake of fast food to ensure that you don't over-indulge in unhealthy foods. These types of foods that have a low nutritional value but high-fat content will fill you up when you eat them, but you will feel the sensation of unsatisfied nauseation after a big meal. This is because, though filling, the food that you have consumed is not nutritious and rather saturated with hidden fats and cholesterol.

Environmental Toxins and Poor Health Habits

We, unfortunately, treat harmful foods as a reward for positive behavior or something we can binge after a tough day or traumatic experience. This type of behavior is far more regularly experienced than most realize. Our society views food as an escape from reality, which can become dangerous when a person gravitates towards unhealthy variants of food. Consider your relationship with food and ask yourself why your habits are what they are... you might be surprised!

What we put into our bodies and what we immediately desire can adversely affect our gut health. Just as the places and people that influence us can have a significant effect on our overall health in later life. These influential factors can start to affect us as early as conception.

Consider why expectant mothers are advised against consuming alcohol, smoking, or ingesting substances such as caffeine or other adverse substances. Our parents' diets, lifestyles, and other lifestyle choices can and will affect our biome in the womb. Their decisions ultimately dictate the bacteria that surrounds and helps to form our guts as we prepare for birth.

Where we are from and the different kinds of cultures that we are raised in will also have a direct impact on our overall health. The foods we ingest from a young age and the quality of the land and air around us dictate our needs as adults. For instance, growing up around places containing heavy lead concentrations can negatively shape our cognitive development, make us averse to certain types of foods, and predispose us to certain types of diseases. Whatever our living situations in early childhood, our bodies will work in overdrive to compensate for an abundance or lack of chemicals that surround and nourish us.

The functions of the brain are interconnected with the digestive operations in your body, and constantly relay messages according to what types of foods have been consumed. Much like the central nervous system oversees our breathing, the digestive system controls digestion during every step of the way, including regulating blood flow to help with absorbing nutrients. Consequently, it is always communicating with the central nervous system for ultimate guidance.

Because there are so many different kinds of medications that can influence the gut, experts have figured out certain medications (like antidepressants) can actually offset our digestive systems and negatively influence our gut bacteria.

Effects of Stress, Anxiety, and Trauma on the Brain and its Supportive Digestive Processes

We must remember that trauma can influence the gut, even when the stomach and intestines aren't directly affected. Consider your body's response to stress and how you physically feel afterward. Do you experience a stomach ache or changes to your digestive tract when something goes wrong? This can occur because our emotional health and gut health are closely reliant on one another.

A study of children who were raised in the foster care system found that children under emotional duress experienced digestive issues, nausea, and vomiting. The study suggested that children reared in households with disruptions in early caregiving were likely to have different gut health factors during their developmental periods when compared to their "healthier" counterparts.

Stress activates the sympathetic and autonomic nervous systems. These two systems being activated at the same time both foster inflammatory responses in the gut. This leads to cortisol production which breaks down the gut lining leading to issues such as leaky gut.[31] The warring chemicals can complicate things, and lead to higher levels of inflammation—which makes the gut more open to attacks. Acute stress can make SIgA (secretory immunoglobulins) less likely to do their job. These immunoglobulins are responsible for fighting bacteria, parasites, and viruses in the intestinal tract.

IgA that is released in the body also helps to boost immunity and to protect your intestines by preventing harmful chemicals from sticking to your intestinal walls. If you're eating a good amount of foods that promote IgA secretion then this helps to block off waste products or highly reactive chemicals from producing irritation and inflammation that can leave the gut barrier open to attack – a so-called 'leaky gut' or 'permeable gut'.

Exercising and eating enough polyunsaturated fatty acids can help to protect a person's body against the onslaught of oxidative stressors and other nutritionally-based problems. Committing time and effort to these two factors can and will increase a person's HDL cholesterol (the good kind) and will aid in the production of needed hormones.

Diet is key for a lot of our long-term health. Eating too much unnecessary fat can lead to systemic inflammation, obesity, promote the development of hypertension, fatten the liver, create a glucose intolerance, and affect one's blood sugar. All of these problems can lead to greater comorbidities along the way and will influence a person's health. Nutrient deficiencies and high sugar can and most likely will lead to increased gut barrier permeability.

It is paramount to remember that your diet can and will influence how you will ultimately function. Unhealthy diets that are filled with high-fat concentrations and low nutritional values may fill you up for a little while. But, the ultimate problems that these types of diets will cause will become greater problems along the way.

Eating an unhealthy diet may be tempting because many people are drawn toward the idea of juicy patties and melted cheese, but the problems that are ultimately incurred from eating these types of foods regularly will become severely problematic in the near future!

Exercise for your Gut!

Exercise is one of the areas in modern life that has become far too neglected in the last several years, which is unfortunate because of all the needed benefits of exercise. We can all stand to be a little bit more active in our lives. Exercise is one of the best ways to boost one's metabolism, lower LDL cholesterol, oxygenate one's brain, and strengthen one's heart muscle.

As it turns out, one of the best ways to lessen your chances of developing a leaky gut or other comorbid symptoms is to exercise regularly. It's apparent how exercise benefits our physical health and improves our overall wellbeing. Thirty minutes of exercise at least four times a week can do wonders for regulating our weight, lowering our heart rates, and improving our blood pressures. Additionally, in the gut, it can reduce inflammation and speed up the interaction between the brain and the rest of the body.

People must take the time to fir physical activity in their day. Because it does allow people to burn unnecessary calories and boost their metabolisms. This physiological boost allows for other healthy processes to take place in the body and brings about healthier adaptations within one's being. Spending half an hour extra every day will start to bring about the desired changes in your body.

Do NOT neglect to take the time to break a sweat every day. There are significant benefits that you will attain if you spend the time forcing yourself to move. This does not mean that you have to become a professional marathon runner in a few days, and you can spend some time every day performing exercises that you actually enjoy.

One of the best types of exercises that can be performed by people of any age group is walking. It may seem simple, but it is effective. Walking is a great way to get moving, and actually enjoy the environment around you. Just because you feel that you may not be fit enough to perform certain exercises, must not deter you from starting somewhere. Getting up and moving is the beginning step for anyone that is trying to get in shape... and we all have to start somewhere.[32]

Controlling Allergies Helps Your Gut

Allergies can become a serious hindrance in anyone's life; you may need to get tested for allergies. Every single person is different, and this means you will have to address different sensitivities. If you are concerned about the effects of allergies in your life and livelihood, then consult with your physician to run a test of different allergens.

Moderate and severe allergies can have a detrimental effect on your life. Food allergies, especially, can lead to chronic inflammation resulting in symptoms such as fatigue, anxiety, and depression. You should determine what mild intolerances affect you so that you can minimize these interactions in your life. If you can afford it, getting a DNA analysis of your stool may give hints to how you can boost your diet to replace the bad bacteria with the good.

Allergies can be life-threatening in certain instances, but it is important to remember that many of these types of allergies can influence the quality of your life. Many of these allergies are worsened by unhealthy diets and the constant introduction of unhealthy additives.

Many allergies that you are facing today can actually be the result of bad eating habits and an unhealthy lifestyle. My patients have seen a remarkable reduction in their allergies after they stopped eating "junk" food and focused on a healthier lifestyle.

This can occur because the gut and the central nervous system communicate very closely. If a person is constantly introducing unhealthy additives into their diets, there will be physiological consequences that can cause their immune systems to be "overactive" and worsen allergic reactions.

If you would like to control your allergies, then altering your diet can be greatly beneficial. Allergies are very irritating (and sometimes life-threatening) part of life, but eating healthy foods and maintaining a healthy lifestyle can help control these unnecessary immune responses.

Foods and Supplements that Benefit the GBA

- **Probiotics** are essential to rebuilding gut health. By definition, they alter and add to the microbiota and microflora in a person's stomach and intestines to the benefit of whoever has ingested them. An example of this that I use in my clinic is is "Megaspore" which contains a healthy blend of multiple probiotics. Megaspore uses a spore form which is not affected by stomach acid like other probiotics.
- **Vitamin A** has been shown to regulate the stability of retinoic acid, which benefits barrier

function and keeps cells tight. It is important to remember, however, that vitamin A is a fat-soluble vitamin and can become toxic if more is taken than the recommended daily dose. Always keep within the daily ranges when taking vitamins.

- **Vitamin D** receptors are extremely important for the gut's barrier to renew cells and regulate the immune function. We do not take in nearly as much vitamin D as we should, on average. It is best to consider taking a vitamin D supplement. That said, if you live in an area that is high in UV rays, then your body will naturally produce vitamin D, and supplements should only be considered in countries in the Northern Hemisphere.

- **Magnesium** can help keep cells tight together and regulate the number of bacteria in the gut and naturally boost the immune system.

- **Omega-3 fatty acids** are important for influencing immune function and inflammation. Ingesting more omega-3 fatty acids can help produce cytokines and antigens in the immune system to help stave off illness and inflammation.

- **Zinc** is greatly imperative in the functioning of the immune system and a zinc deficiency can break down tight cell connections and create sensitive areas in the gut. This can create more openings in the gut when the mucosal linings are exposed to possible stressors such as alcohol.

- **Fermented foods** are greatly beneficial to a person's overall health and well-being because of the way that they can boost the immune system because of their antioxidant concentrations. That said, it is important to carefully research which fermented foods are safe to consume without causing unnecessary strain on other of your bodily organs. Some include kimchi, sauerkraut, and miso.

- **ADP** (adeno-diphosphates) are energy molecules that are broken down from ATP (adeno-triphosphates) during metabolic processes and can be found as a natural supplement extracted from herbs like oregano and dried thyme. These herbs release this energy molecule when pulverized in a way that allows the capsule that can slow the growth of parasitic organisms in the bacteria.

- This energy molecule doesn't normally have to be taken from other sources, because they are primarily produced from the foods that we eat. It is just important that you remember to eat healthy foods to maintain this type of energy output.

- **Include spices into your diet**: Thyme, cloves, anise, betulina, and dill are just a few spices that can serve as effective antimicrobials. You can incorporate these spices into your daily cooking for impressive and tasty benefits.[33]

TIP: Support the Gut, Support the Brain

In modern times, medicine is 'evidence-based' which means that the modern approach is systematic and careful, based on observation, feedback, and carefully interpreting your data. This approach to our personal healing is the one that tends to work best for us at home too. In that spirit, I recommend journaling your day to day diet and food choices. Recording your foods, your moods, the things you try, and how they affect you is the best way to check on what works and what doesn't.

Documenting how you feel day-to-day, recording what you eat, what you took in terms of supplements, how clear your thinking was, and how you felt (moods) on each day is a very helpful way to see patterns over time, and can be very useful to you (and your doctor) to help tailor your health choices to suit your needs perfectly.

The process shouldn't take much of your time, just note the date, the time of entry, and the essential information – 10 minutes in the evening at most, any longer and your journal might be including unnecessary information.

When your lifestyle starts to evolve into a healthier routine, it will be necessary for you to *keep improving* your lifestyle into healthier and healthier alternatives. This will take some adjustments, but you will quickly come to see the wisdom of this approach. Negative catch-22 downward health spirals aren't the only kinds of health spirals out there. The very same mechanisms that perpetuate ever degenerating health can also be reversed and turned to your favor. Upward spiraling health builds on prior upward spiraling health. Eventually, a plateau will be reached and then your journaling comes in handy because it will let you see what behavior has the most impact, and what behavior can be left behind.

Recording your experiences and interventions can help you measure the success that different kinds of habits and behavior are actually having – it is an important way to measure your success objectively. This is especially needed when reclaiming your brain since your cognitions might be biased because of the poor state of your brain health. In that case, seeing the facts objectively written down will help you keep the right perspective.

Always ask yourself whether you could have done a little bit more for your body and brain today. For example, you know about certain fruits, nuts, and foods that are packed with potent brain-enhancing compounds, so you could always be asking whether you considered adding extra berries, vegetables, lean meats, and fish to your meals – this keeps your thinking proactive, positive, and engaged with the beneficial facts and methods in this book.

With that attitude, and a little diligence, new habits turn into unconscious ways of being healthy automatically – imagine what happens when you are already healthy and you begin to exercise your willpower and choices over a healthy domain, then it really does become a matter of "the sky is the limit". Measuring your success is very rewarding, and doing it helps to keep perspective when an occasional bad day comes along amidst countless good days – keep yourself motivated, buoyant, and focused – be smart, do it for yourself and reap the rewards you most definitely deserve.

Improve Your Diet, Improve Your Gut, Improve Your Brain

When we are injured, our body falls back on its natural defenses that are there to protect us. If we are constantly eating foods that are injuring us, we constantly activate our immune system.

Our culture or society doesn't seem to really foster or support healthy attitudes toward foods and eating. Often we are taught that when it comes to eating, quantity is more important than quality. The most available food is laden with fats, salt, and sugar. These items, while vital in small doses, are seldom found naturally in the food we eat, nor in such high quantities as is found in prepared commercial food.

The solution lies in a Mediterranean diet, which places an emphasis on complex carbohydrates in the form of fruits and vegetables. Additionally, it places an emphasis on lean protein in the form of chicken, seafood, or poultry, if it utilizes meats at all.

The worst part about our diets as Americans is that we consume excessive amounts of sodium and sugar. Sodium, most commonly found in salt, can in excess make us more likely to experience cardiovascular issues. The average serving of sodium recommended by experts is just over a teaspoon. If we are not adding salt to our meals at will, we are eating them as preservatives in frozen food items, addictive amounts in restaurant items, and in red meat.

Consuming sodium in your diet is actually more dangerous than people realize. Yes, salt is needed to flavor and preserve foods, but it can cause problems regarding hypertension. According to chemistry and physiology, water will always follow sodium through a permeable channel because the positive electrolyte (sodium) ions attract the negative oxygen ions in the water molecules and the water flows where the salt is.

The same process happens in a person's blood vessels when they consume sodium in their diets. The sodium becomes absorbed into the bloodstream, and because the sodium concentration in the blood vessels has increased, the sodium starts to draw fluid out of the body cells and into the bloodstream. This causes a rise in blood pressure. Research has found that by simply cutting out salt from one's diet, a person can significantly lower their blood pressure without the use of any medications.

Salt is needed but it can be detrimental if used incorrectly. The same principle applies to sugar. Sugar, as we discussed in previous chapters, can worsen our chances of developing diabetes, and should be used only in moderation. Remember, that diabetes does predispose one to develop forms of dementia later on in life. Sometimes, certain sacrifices are worthwhile to make for future gain.

Ultimately, the hippocampus, the memory center, is at stake when we follow a western diet paired with a sedentary lifestyle because it keeps needing to secrete copious amounts of stress hormone which will cause damage to the body and the hippocampus itself.

Finally, if you want to still enjoy tasty food, but not worry about harming your body in the process, then it is necessary to follow meal plans according to the Mediterranean diet. The Mediterranean diet is essential in blocking off the amount of fat prevalent in our food, and because you will be consuming healthy fats and other nutritious goodness, you won't likely crave unhealthy foods after you switch over to this meal plan. Eating too much fat can also raise our blood pressure and make us more susceptible to cardiovascular illnesses because of the increased levels of LDL cholesterol. The Mediterranean diet advises us to substitute fatty items for leaner solutions that pack more protein than fat.

Following the Mediterranean diet helps us promote the brain because it allows the brain to absorb more antioxidants. It also promotes the growth of nitric oxide, which leads to the creation and repairing of cells. Paired with physical activity and intellectual activity, it leads to better brain health, better cognitive performance, and cognitive preserves.

By promoting these forms of nutrients, we naturally eat less unnecessary sodium, because we have provided our bodies with the essential nutrients needed to thrive. [34]

A Mediterranean Meal Example

If you want to fully embrace a healthier lifestyle, then you are going to have to learn to enjoy being in the kitchen. If you cook for yourself, then you can personally control how much nutrition you can pack into a meal, and how much of the "bad stuff" you can forgo. Besides, many people that start to experiment in the kitchen start to discover that they actually enjoy cooking.

Being in the kitchen allows for great family time or quality spousal time, and you can start to practice some impressive culinary skills. When you have decided to adopt a more Mediterranean type of diet plan, then you will have to change the way that you shop.

You can't go into shops any longer and browse all of the aisles that are filled with food items that you know you struggle with. If you are trying to get healthy, then avoid walking in the path of temptation. Go in with a shopping list and head straight for the aisles that you know you will need to go down. This may be difficult in the beginning, but it will become easier with time.

This recipe is simple, but it is delicious. Remember that you are trying to pack as many nutrients into your plate, without affecting the overall caloric value of your dish. The dish of "creamed spinach stuffed chicken breasts" will make anyone's day. The reason I am including this recipe is that it's easy to make and because spinach is such a healthy green (that benefits from being cooked) it is a great one to eat regularly.

A simple Meal Example: Healthy Stuffed Mediterranean Chicken Breasts on Brown Rice

Ingredients and Cooking Methods

I am writing down this recipe to serve two adults, but it can be easily adjusted to feed more people if you so desire. Grab two large, boneless, skinless chicken breasts and slice them down one of the sides so that you can easily tease it open. (Don't cut all the way through, because it will make the stuffing process rather difficult.)

Once the above is done, season the breasts with a touch of salt, black pepper, and dried oregano on both outer sides as well as on the inside of the central spaces. Place them aside and wilt/lightly heat 200 grams of fresh spinach in a pot with a teaspoon of extra virgin olive oil - until completely wilted. Add a cup of Greek yogurt to the spinach and season to taste. Crumb a block of low-fat feta cheese into the creamy concoction and set aside.

Preheat your oven to 400 degrees Fahrenheit (just under 205 degrees Celsius). While you are waiting for the oven to heat up, you can stuff the creamed spinach into the cavities on the breasts and then close the sides of the slit with toothpicks.

Place the chicken breasts in the preheated oven for about 30 minutes, or cook all the way through. Serve the stuffed breasts on a bed of brown rice with a small green salad on the side.

This dish is simple, yet delicious and may become one of the firm favorites in your household.

Food for the Brain Tip #1:

Learn to enjoy cooking and you will reap the benefits of preparing healthy meals. Don't continue to eat unhealthy products because they are going to take their toll in the long-run. Remember, "if you eat inflammation, you become inflammation!"

Food for the Brain Tip #2:

Consume foods that are high in omega-3 fatty acids regularly to protect your heart and brain. Fortunately, this is rather easy when you move onto a Mediterranean diet.

7

SLEEP, EXERCISE, STRESS & ANXIETY

Exercise for Body, Brain, and Happiness

When we exercise, we raise our heart rate, temperature, and circulate more oxygen throughout the body. Increased oxygen levels generate increased energy (exercise generates energy!), and helps to repair our mitochondria (the little energy factories of the body found inside each cell) and the metabolic mechanisms that produce energy.

Improving mitochondrial health and regenerating mitochondrial based metabolic systems improves every single system in the body!

In one shot we can improve our total health and wellbeing simply and decisively. Amazingly, when our mitochondria function optimally then they can take toxic free radicals out of our tissues and convert them into energy – could there be anything more beneficial?[1] [2] [3]

Aside from better oxygenation, improving blood flow and raising temperature serves to effectively move metabolic by-products (and waste products) out of problem areas. Sweating is a good example of the supreme efficiency and intelligence latent in the body. Sweating keeps us cool when we are hot, but the body also eliminates waste products in sweat – nothing is wasted, ever.

The by-products affected by exercise can include plaques, lactic acid, free radicals, allergens (particles that induce immune reactions and inflammation), and many more. [4]

Insights generated by research into exercise have discovered that exercise releases cytokines like interleukin-6 (IL-6). IL-6 transforms carbohydrates into glucose, reduces tumor growth rates, and stimulates the production of anti-inflammatory cytokines as well as aiding in the breakdown of lipids. Too much IL-6 in the body is associated with lipid aggregation (not great for the heart) but this effect is always more than adequately offset by the increased removal of waste products from the body.[5]

Exercise definitely improves the blood vessels and circulatory system as a whole. [6] Not only does exercise improve basic biological functioning, but time and again exercise has been linked with better cognitive performance – people who exercise think better. No one single mechanism has been linked to the increase in cognitive function, instead, the increased mental benefit is thought to be due to a total improvement in multiple factors affecting brain function; factors like better blood flow, readily available energy, and a diminishment in factors contributing to brain damage. Think (!) about it this way, if your body is efficient, energy sufficient, and waste product free then it is likely that your wakeful states of consciousness would be perfused with greater clarity and attention.[7] [8] [9] [10]

Excitingly, exercise helps grow new nerve cells, and thus supports neuroplasticity – the ability for our brain to regrow and reconnect itself in different ways as it learns and adapts to the environment around it.[11]

> *"The neuroprotective, cardio-protective, metabolic supporting, general health-protecting properties of exercise are the undeniable guiding justification for stating that one should exercise for total health and well-being."*

Exercise in some form has proven to be beneficial for cardiovascular disease (treatment and prevention)[12], cancer[13], diabetes[14] [15] [16], obesity[17], Alzheimer's disease[18] [19], Parkinson's disease[20] [21], insomnia[22] [23] [24]*, and just about every other ailment ever recorded (ever)!* [25] [26]

Types of Exercise

There are different kinds of exercise and each has different benefits and drawbacks. I have already shown that exercise is beneficial, always! But, exercise for the brain comes in three different types viz. cardiovascular (cardio), strength, and brain exercises for brain function.

Cardiovascular (cardio) Exercises

There is no excuse for not performing cardio exercises, including old age. It is important to find cardio exercises that you are comfortable with, and capable of performing without inflicting any injuries on your body.

If you are young and would like to get back into an exercising routine as you had in school, then there are several variations that you include to keep you entertained and make you fit in the process.

In the beginning stages of exercising, you are going to feel like you are dying...don't worry, this is normal–especially if you haven't done it for a while. It will take a few weeks of continuous exercise to get to the place where you don't feel like your heart is about to burst out of your chest.

The trick here is variation. Don't fall into the trap of performing the same types of exercises day in and day out, because you will get tired of the monotony and start making up excuses not to exercise. Throw different things into the mix to keep it enjoyable. There are many cardio exercises that you can partake in to keep yourself from growing bored. There are cardio variations like skipping, swimming, cycling, that you can introduce into your routine for variation and different muscle activations.

A friend of mine used to run a lot during his younger days, and he told me that he hated running in the beginning because he always felt like he was dying when he attempted it. But as his fitness grew, so did his boredom. He soon realized that if he didn't run with someone else, he wouldn't run at all because he had no one to talk to. He eventually told me about his internal rule that he gave to himself about running, which was if a person could maintain an in-depth conversation while running and not sounding out of breath, then it would be necessary to throw in some more difficult exercises.

Now, this is doable for younger people, but you may read this and think to yourself that there is no way that you are going to perform intensive cardio exercises. Fortunately, you don't have to. This book is not designed to tell you to drop a certain amount of pounds in a month, but it is telling you to exercise to protect your brain.

Research has found that walking is actually the best cardio-vascular exercise to help ward off the effects of cognitive illnesses. The reason for this is two-fold. First, the actual movement of walking allows for adequate lung expansion and oxygenation of the blood. (This, in turn, increases the amount of oxygen that goes to the brain). Second, the environmental stimuli around a person work excellently to maintain neural pathways. So, actually walking around and looking at the birds and the trees can help protect the brain and how it functions.

An old patient of mine developed Alzheimer's later on in life, and although he was a very pleasant man, I could see that the onset of this disease was taking a toll on his wife and their marriage. I asked them about their living habits, and how his symptoms were progressing. His Alzheimer's development wasn't as rapid as I thought it would be, and he still remembered many aspects of his life.

After assessing him I asked him what exercises he performed because even though he was old, he did look very fit for his age. His wife informed me that one thing that he remembered to do every day was to go for long walks. It was a habit that he formed very early on in his life, and it definitely slowed the progression of his illness.

I still keep in contact with this patient and assess him on a semi-regular basis, and even though there is no cure for this cognitive illness, his healthy eating habits and daily forms of exercise have slowed the progression of his Alzheimer's.

Strength Exercises

It is important for people who are trying to maintain their overall health to spend some time a few times a week on strength training. These exercises are not actually meant to give you a nice body (which they may in any case), but rather to protect your brain and keep it healthy.

Strength exercises work different muscle groups in the body. They naturally boost the metabolism and increase the amount of oxygen moving around in the body, because a person's lung capacity does become larger the more strength training they do. The reason for this is because it takes repetitions of deep breathing to be able to lift certain weights.

If you are worried that I am about to tell you to sign up at your nearest gym, then you don't have to be alarmed. Body-weight exercises work excellently to strengthen one's body, oxygenate the brain, and boost metabolism.

All of the bodyweight exercises that will benefit you, you can perform in your home or in your garden. Push-ups, pull-ups, and planking will greatly strengthen your body and increase the amount of air that you can breathe in one breath, and increase the amount of oxygen that will become available in your body.

Strength exercises are great additions to your exercise routines and you will reap the benefits of these types of exercises if you regularly incorporate them.

Brain Exercises

You need to view your brain as a muscle that needs to be exercised. Of course, you won't be able to do bicep curls with your mind, but you do need to find ways to train your brain. These days, physical exercise has become a rather neglected pastime for many people who do not seem to be able to find the time to do it in our busy, hectic, day-to-day modern grind – it is unfortunate, and a little saddening too, that the same could be said for many people about them actually using their brains. That is not to say that stupidity or lack of careful thoughtful mindful attitudes are becoming commonplace (they might be), but that rather people seldom think to exercise their brains like they know they should any other muscles in the body. We need to think, particularly about things we haven't thought about before. We need to learn new skills and concepts every year just to keep the neurons in our brains happy, healthy, and strong.

It is far too easy for people to sit and act as a vegetable in front of the TV and not think. This can become a dangerous habit because the brain needs to be exercised to stay healthy. There are many different kinds of exercises that people can perform to actually strengthen their brains. It may sound like a weird concept, but actually spending time and forcing your brain to think and learn new concepts, keeps the serotonin and acetylcholine levels in the brain at a healthy constant which will maintain healthy communication between the cells and maintain neural connections.

Brain exercising can come down to any type of event that helps you think. Certain board games, like chess and "Risk," require a lot of strategizing and can allow a person's mind to maintain neural connections. The reason why this is important is that these connections are very elastic at birth and making new pathways and connections is very easy for young people. This elastic trait, unfortunately, slows down with age, and it becomes more difficult for adults to make new neural pathways. This is why it is far easier for young children to learn new languages than their adult counterparts.

Neural plasticity is a blessing, and even though it may decrease with time, it is still vitally important to train your brain and keep the connections that you have established healthy. That said, it does not mean that adults can't learn new concepts in later years, but it does take significantly more work.

Training your brain takes time, and as with other forms of exercise you will need to take time out of your day to commit to brain exercises. But, this is where you can use your imagination. Reading, drawing, writing, playing Sudoku, crosswords, and solving math problems are great ways to help your neurons communicate with one another.

It is vitally important for people to exercise their brains and learn new concepts. You may not be able to make new neural connections in advanced years of age, but you will be able to maintain the ones that you have established and kept them healthy. Making these new healthy habits in your life will bring about remarkable changes and you will be able to protect your brain from any unfortunate cognitive illnesses that do sneak up on people as they get older.

Incorporating new eating habits, physical exercises, and mental exercises into your daily routine will protect your brain. If you are younger and busy reading this book, then you have the time and opportunity now to become healthier and protect your brain before developing illnesses later on in life. If you are older and have already started experiencing some cognitive symptoms, then you can still make changes with these healthy habits and slow down any unfortunate cognitive developments.

Cleanse Your Mind –Stress, Happiness & Brain Health

High levels of chronic stress are related to elevated levels of cortisol (a stress hormone) and heightened over activation of the amygdala – a brain region responsible for fear responses, base drives, and memory.

The most compelling link between stress and brain health and performance is that stress is directly linked to heart disease and our heart and blood vessels are one of the key factors in supporting our brain health. Not only that, but people definitely underperform when they are too stressed, heart, and blood vessels aside.

The link between stress and heart problems was shown clearly by a study that linked increased activity in the amygdala with increased inflammation of the arteries (!) – this is a really bad outcome for people with Alzheimer's disease, Parkinson's, and migraines, let alone people trying to think clearly.[27] [28] But this is not the only research finding showing that stress is bad for our brains and hearts, numerous other studies are showing the vast ill effects that stress has on our body and our quality of life. For example, the far-reaching effects of chronic stress also affect fertility, *sleep, appetite, mood, behavior, memory, and cognitive function extremely negatively!*[29]

People who are stressed often make use of coping behaviors such as changes in diet – often too high carbohydrate, high-fat convenience comfort foods. Finally, chronic stress is linked to high blood pressure (hypertension) and other blood and heart and brain changes that are known to correlate with elevated risk for heart disease, decreased mental performance, poor health outcomes, and a much higher likelihood of developing a chronic degenerative disease. [30] [31]

Thus, it should be clear that stress is a key player in bad health and affects our quality of life at a fundamental level. [32]

People suffering from chronic stress are also more likely to develop depression. Our sense of happiness, satisfaction, drive, and reward is thought to be regulated by neurotransmitters in the brain. If you think back to chapter one of this book, you will remember that neurotransmitters are essentially tiny little chemical messengers that trigger body systems and regulate behavior and mood – you could call them molecules of emotion, regulation, and thinking.

The key neurotransmitters involved in the abovementioned psychological states are serotonin, melatonin, dopamine, oxytocin, testosterone, and some others. Dopamine is considered to be linked to pleasure and feelings of bliss and reward, whilst serotonin and melatonin regulate our waking and sleep cycles as well as our moods (happy/sad). A full discussion of the body's neuropsychological chemistry, regulating systems, and modulating effects are way beyond the scope of this book, but keep this in mind – there are chemicals associated with our states of consciousness, and disruptions in their levels can induce depression, anxiety, and other symptoms.

So, the core chemical messenger responsible for stress in the body is cortisol whilst the core messenger for happiness is serotonin – you can consider these two chemicals as being 'psychological' opposites of each other. Whilst this represents an overly simplified view it is enough to understand how to improve happiness and decrease stress – both of which are correlated with heart disease.

How do we get our stress under control? Well, two approaches make the most sense. First, it is important to realize that in general, if we are feeling happy then that directly decreases our chronic or acute stress levels – cortisol levels decrease, and serotonin increases. On the other hand, we can directly decrease our cortisol levels by making a conscious effort to relax in conjunction with supplementation to promote the biological mechanisms of relaxation as well as manage our human interactions skillfully. [33] [34]

Strategies to Decrease Stress & Improve Happiness

Strike a Pose at Work

Surprisingly our body language actually affects the levels of neurotransmitters in the body. Power poses have been shown to not only decrease cortisol levels but also increase testosterone levels and increase our sense of power, satisfaction, and happiness.

Two studies showed the effects of stress and dominance on hormones in the body in social situations. The two studies reported that testosterone and cortisol are linked together and that they rise and fall together depending on perceived dominance versus submission. Thus our stress (cortisol) and dominance (testosterone) levels are directly based on our perceptions of our apparent success in social situations.[35] It has been found that simply adopting 'power poses' alone or in social settings seems to 'trick' the body into feeling more powerful and dominant – decreasing cortisol and raising testosterone levels significantly.[36] Simply by assuming a simple pose for one minute, a person can decrease stress and become happier – amazing.[37] [38] Adopting more submissive poses is correlated with higher cortisol and lower testosterone – sometimes by as much as 25%. Three key power stances researched in the literature are 1) Placing both palms face down on a table a shoulder-width apart; 2) Hands behind the head and sitting cross-legged in a chair. 3) Standing with feet slightly apart with arms akimbo. After these studies many other postures have been tried and identified to be extremely effective – most stances are modeled after primate postures or the body language of 'successful' people. [39]

Eat Food for Serotonin

It stands to reason that if the body has plenty of the materials it requires to produce serotonin then it will be able to produce it when it needs to. Now ensuring that one has sufficient serotonin precursors in the body does not guarantee that the brain will activate more serotonin pathways. However, having sufficient precursors will ensure that should the brain increase serotonin production and activation then it will not be short of what it requires. What substances are used in serotonin production? The following are some of the better known and easily available supplements supporting serotonin function in the body:

- Vitamin B6 & B12 supplements
- Tryptophan
- Vitamin B6 & Vitamin B12 rich foods such as bananas, avocados, and legumes.
- Tryptophan rich foods such as red meats, chicken, turkey, nuts, and eggs.

Exercise...again!

Once again the benefits of mild aerobic exercise are potent – they protect the brain and heart and every other major system and organ of the body. Mild aerobic exercise has been shown to stimulate serotonin production as well as many other neurotransmitters and hormones. For more detail on exercise refer to the section on exercise just a bit earlier in this very chapter.

Good Regular Sleep

Not sleeping is related to very poor health outcomes including directly contributing to the causes and risk factors of poor brain health, heart disease, stress, depression, and many other problems besides. To make the point extremely clear the following health complications are associated with insomnia:

- Insomnia leads to higher levels of cortisol, epinephrine, and other stress hormones.[40] [41]
- Raised levels of cortisol lead to increased weight gain, poor immune functioning, and a heightened risk of diabetes and osteoporosis.[42] [43] [44]
- Insomnia increases inflammation in the body because of increased secretion of hormones like interleukin-6 (IL-6) and tumor necrosis factor-alpha (TNF–α). Chronically elevated levels of IL-6 and TNF-α are linked to arthritis, IBS (inflammatory bowel syndrome), and heart disease.[45]
- Insomnia makes us more sensitive to pain and therefore worsens conditions associated with

chronic pain.[46] Examples include arthritis and fibromyalgia. What is more, chronic pain can prevent sleep which in turn can cause insomnia which leads to chronic pain, and so on. A horrifying catch-22 cycle of painful sleep disturbance. This is very bad news for people with migraines, and it is very difficult to perform mentally when you are awash with little aches and pains, let alone chronic levels of intense pain and inflammation.

- Adults who do not get enough sleep on a chronic basis have up to four times the risk of stroke than those who usually get a good night's sleep – a sign of high stress, bad consequences for the heart, and difficulty managing daily life.[47]
- Finally and most disturbingly, adults with insomnia have an increased risk of death due to any cause.

Sleep is an extremely important aspect of health and overall quality of life. Studies indicate that between seven and eight hours of sleep per night in a regular pattern is best for maintaining optimal health.[48] [49]

Being Mindful – Meditation for the Brain and Heart

Meditation is the intentional mindful activity of focusing on present awareness and resting consciousness naturally in an uncontrived fashion. Many studies show the benefits of meditation for our heart health, stress reduction, better memory, and overall cognitive function.

Sitting meditation with controlled breathing bears all the hallmarks of good heart health. Breathing slows along with heart rate, whilst stress levels decrease in response to imminent relaxation. The following benefits have been recorded in the research literature:

- A Harvard study showed that meditation/mindfulness practice enabled the regrowth of grey matter in the brain over 8 weeks. [50]

- Another study showed that meditation was able to decrease ADHD symptoms whilst increasing attention span. [51]

- Further findings showed that meditation reduces systolic blood pressure. [52]

- The American Heart Association (AHA) states unequivocally that meditation reduces blood pressure [53].

- The long term effects of stress reduction due to meditation have been correlated with a 23% decrease in all causes of mortality. [54]

- Meditation can change genes involved in regulating life span – stimulating telomerase production. [55]

In short, meditation is an extremely skillful method of managing stress, improving attention, decreasing blood pressure, and promoting all-around robust health. Meditating increases your expected lifespan, helps your brain to regrow and heal and stay healthy, and it decreases heart disease risk.

If you would like to try meditation or mindfulness practice then you can try the simple technique of 'counting your breath'.

There are no hard and fast rules and the general principle is to sit quietly in the manner you are accustomed to. Make sure you are comfortable and maintain a clear awake awareness – don't fall asleep. Then pay attention to your own breathing watching the in and out breaths without attempting to control or alter the breath in any way. Count the breaths up to ten e.g. in-breath 1; out-breath 2; in-breath 3.........out-breath 10. Once you reach the end of out-breath-10 then begin the count again at in-breath-1 etc.

When people first start meditating, they usually discover that five minutes feels like an extremely long time - almost an eternity. But as familiarity with it develops, people can maintain a calm relaxed meditation session for 30 minutes to an hour, or longer.

Furthermore, and this may come as a surprise to many people, they often find it difficult to just calmly focus on the breath. Most people find that instead of just simply focusing on their breathing their mind tends to wander off into thoughts, emotions, and mental images or fantasies. This is completely normal; it just shows you how busy your inner mental world actually is.

When you notice that you have wandered off mentally just calmly bring yourself back to your breath and begin the count again. There is no right way to do the practice – the only advice is to relax and enjoy it. It is in relaxing and enjoying that we decrease stress and increase happiness. This is the main reason for mentioning meditation in this book.

If you enjoy the above meditation you may want to explore it further. There are many other great sources of information such as books, audio CDs, binaural beats, hypnosis, and even meditation teachers that can help you to explore your minds more deeply. Exploring meditation can also potentially lead to a deep appreciation of some of the rich and long-standing history of contemplative cultures from all around the world, as well as the techniques that they have employed for exploring the mind and body for many thousands of years.

As for relaxing binaural beats and other "kick-start methods" there is also a substantial body of research showing their beneficial effects on our stress, happiness, heart health, and brain health.[56] Meditation has the potential to help develop certain meditative stability to your mental states which really helps us to navigate our daily lives in a more skillful and response-able way.[57]

Our reactions to stress and traumatic events have made us excellent survivors over the millennia. We are equipped with fight-or-flight responses that trigger different chemicals in the brain and help us rapidly make decisions. The stress response is great for life-or-death situations that our distant ancestors often found themselves facing. However, it's not so great for every single troubling occurrence in our lives.

The constant, high-stress environments that practically all people live in nowadays are causing a myriad of health problems. One of the main problems with being constantly stressed is that it can cause unnecessary inflammation. This occurs because, in times of intense stress, the body starts to release cortisol (the stress hormone), because the body perceives that it may be in trouble and secretes this hormone to try and fight the current stressor. This is not a problem when a person is actually in danger but the long term it can lead to depression, anxiety, weight gain, inflammation, chronic fatigue, heart problems, chronic illnesses of many kinds, and poor mental performance and health.

Depression is fueled by chronic inflammation that occurs in our brains. Inflammatory messages trigger responses in our hypothalamus, which collects information on the body's well-being. The hypothalamus signals to the adrenal glands to produce cortisol and DHEA, two stress hormones. This can lead to cortisol dissolving your gut lining because it is rich in amino acids. This happens to fuel the stress response but leaves no resources for important neurotransmitters which play a role in mental stability.[58]

We all face stress at some point in our daily lives. However, those who suffer more frequently from stress may be experiencing anxiety-related illnesses. Anxiety is the most common form of mental health problem, materializing in many ways — one of which is depression. Around 40 million U.S. adults suffer from anxiety disorders annually, and many of them choose to seek professional help. Within this realm is depression, which is responsible for keeping more people from work than any other disorder.

Depression may be caused by several different emotional problems, but some physiological problems may cause depressive episodes too. Depression may be caused by imbalances in the thyroid gland. If you are worried that you might be depressed because of hormone imbalances, then it may be necessary to get tested by your doctor. You should be tested for reverse T3, free serum thyroxine, thyroid-stimulating hormone, anti-thyroglobulin antibodies, and anti-thyroid peroxidase antibodies. Many physicians only test for thyroid-stimulating hormone, which is a disservice to you and your health because there are other precipitating factors and hormone imbalances that can lead to depression.

Other deficiencies can cause depression, and many of them have to do with vitamins and minerals. Imbalances in diet and nutritional intake can result in unexplainable mood swings. One of the minerals that can cause depression in a person if it's lacking is zinc. If you are feeling more blue than normal, you may have a zinc deficiency. This simple mineral plays a vital role in the body from the immune system to one of the major precursors in hormonal development.

Anxiety and depression are both manageable when we focus on the factors we can control and optimize for our own well-being. These include proper diet, exercise, and stress management which are by far the most inexpensive treatment comparatively. Many people choose medication to fight the symptoms of depression, however, this only covering up the symptoms and not addressing the root cause. While everyone copes differently, it is important to become educated about the different treatment modalities available.[59]

Strong Brain Tip for Moods #1:

Anxiety can come in many forms, whether spiritually, mentally, emotionally, or physically. Thus, different types of treatment may be best for certain forms of anxiety. Try a variety of self-care methods to see what best suits your needs. Great examples include journaling, meditation, mindful creative coloring-in, and exercise.

Strong Brain Tip for Moods #2:

Incorporate activities you enjoy into your day to boost both your attitude and mood. Don't stick to activities that don't bring you pleasure – drop what doesn't serve you. When you start exercising, start at your level and slowly adjust your regime as your fitness improves – no need to 'push it' just a simple consistent daily effort is more than enough. Enjoy your self-care, looking after yourself is not a chore, it is a supreme pleasure. If you approach it in this way you will make it a life-long habit, and that is all that is required for immense beneficial change to happen to you.

Environmental Harmony

The environment that you are in will obviously affect you both emotionally and physically. Reducing exposure to environmental toxins can reduce stress on the nervous system to allow for healing.

Living in an environment that is unhealthy (due to unnatural stressors or even dangerous toxins) will take a large toll on you. It is important to remember that environmental toxins can create severe neurological issues, even when a person's diet is fine. It doesn't help to eat healthily, but you are still exposed to other toxins every day that are harming you in the process.

If you are still experiencing issues after changing your diet, consult with a medical professional to get lab testing done. There may be underlying problems that need to be addressed to help you get healthy again.

If you are worried about the overall influence of the environment that you are in, then you may need to try distancing yourself from that particular environment. If you can afford to vacation, do so. Or, try spending a day or two in a different home or try working from a different place.

If during the time away, your symptoms improve, then you may have found your answer about what is affecting your physical condition and brain health. It is important to note, that if you do suspect that there are areas in your work or home environment that are actually harming you, then you will have to take action before the symptoms worsen.

There are many signs that you may have to look out for if you're worried about environmental toxins, but there are other factors that can be affecting your brain health without actually affecting you with literal toxins.

The Stressful Workplace

Another aspect that can greatly interfere with your brain health is being part of a working environment that is too stressful. As I mentioned earlier, being in an overly stressed environment will release large amounts of stress (fight or flight) hormones on a far too frequent basis. This, in turn, will cause other problems in your body and you will start to put on weight.

The other downside to this is the fact that the hippocampus and adrenal glands will eventually become severely depleted because they will be secreting such large amounts of stress hormones too regularly.

There are myriad health problems that can occur with being in an environment that is too stressful. If you think that you are in an environment that is too stressful and that it is affecting the health of your body and brain, then it will be necessary to weigh up the options of staying in that environment. If, however, you can't escape that environment, then it may be necessary to find other ways to cope with the stress to maintain your brain's overall health.

Healthy Environment Tip:

If you can't escape emotional stress, then you can develop and maintain a regular mindfulness practice or two to help regulate your mood and emotions. Even if you are in a position in which you cannot escape. Many find solace through journaling or even cataloging the things they have accomplished throughout the day. Some have found that meditating for as little as five minutes per day has increased their mood exponentially. There are many different formats of journals, as well as a plethora of mindfulness tools, that are freely available. Try these tools and figure out what works best for you.

8

NATURAL SUPPLEMENTS & SUPER-FOODS TO HEAL, PROTECT, AND BOOST YOUR BRAIN

What follows is a comprehensive review of the awesome power that nature has to impact your brain positively. Please bear in mind that although these supplements are extremely good for your brain, often the reason that they have such good effects on brain health and function is that they are extremely good for other important systems in the body. Basically, every potent natural tool that I describe in this chapter is really good for the body in some way, particularly when it supports a critical factor of brain health like the heart or immune system.

The above being said, then all that remains to say before I proudly share the tools in this chapter with you is that each entry in this chapter is a short description of a naturally derived food, vitamin, supplement, herb, compound, or other natural sources that have good scientific evidence supporting its power to benefit the body and brain's health and performance -these are the supplements that you should be considering with a healthcare professional to heal, maintain, and boost your brain.

Naturally Derived Nutraceuticals & Supplementation

Luteolin

Luteolin is a member of a group of plant compounds (flavonoids) that has shown significant beneficial results for Alzheimer's disease, Parkinson's, and many neurological disorders. Scientists suspect that Luteolin works by activating your energy metabolism pathways (AMP) and helping the energy factories of the body (called "mitochondria") keep in balance. Luteolin was shown to protect cognitive functions in the brain linked to memory and other performance areas. It managed to do this because it was seen to have beneficial effects on the particular area of the brain called the "hippocampus" which is known to be linked to memory.[1]

Luteolin managed to reduce the toxicity caused by excessive copper[2], as well as prevent the build-up of amyloid-beta peptides into plaques (great for Alzheimer's disease). In another study, luteolin extract protected the brain against trauma-induced injuries which share many of the same pathologies as Alzheimer's disease.[3]

Coenzyme Q10 (Co-Q10)

Co-enzyme Q10 is a compound that works with energy production in the body (ATP, the chemical 'currency' of energy used by the body. It has been suggested for use in the treatment of brain disorders (particularly Alzheimer's) due to its many antioxidant properties.[4][5]

Coenzyme Q10 proved effective at reducing beta-amyloid plaque deposits and overproduction of amyloid-beta building blocks.[6] Another study showed that Coenzyme Q10 had effects in the hippocampus (a brain region linked to memory), and resulted in smarter mice with better performance in tests.[7] People with Alzheimer's, Parkinson's, and other neurodegenerative diseases are much more likely to have deficiencies or deficits in their Co-Q10 levels compared to healthy individuals.[8]

No doubt about it, Co-Q10 is a great candidate supplement to boost mental performance and stabilize energy production in the body.

B Vitamins

A decreased level of B Vitamins has been linked to many brain problems including Alzheimer's disease and many others – in fact, vitamin B deficiency is acknowledged as a potential risk factor for developing Alzheimer's disease.[9] B Vitamins, when in their active, natural forms, have been shown to prevent the rate at which brains atrophy. Furthermore, they improve cognition indirectly.[10] [11] Vitamin B literally helps you to think and process information better.

The B vitamins also impact our stress hormones, levels of anxiety, depression, and generally affect the heart and blood vessels positively – all factors that are critical to having a super performing brain. Vitamin-B lowers homocysteine levels (homocysteine is a blood marker for stress) which are also an associated risk factor for Alzheimer's and heart disease – Homocysteine levels were used to accurately predict the occurrence of Alzheimer's in aging men, the more they had, the higher the chance.[12]

Interestingly, synthetic derivatives of various B vitamins (e.g. folic acid), did not help to reduce Alzheimer's disease symptoms and did not act to prevent or slow the onset and progression of chronic brain illnesses at all.[13] So, this means that we should try to get natural forms of the following B vitamins since those are the ones that have evidence to support that they actually make a big difference to your brain health.

One very important thing to note is that the B-vitamins tend to synergize with each other. This means that if you take supplements to get high doses of B-vitamins you will increase their effects by taking a 'family' of different B-vitamins. This is highly recommended and I encourage you to get a vitamin-B complex multivitamin supplement that has each of the specific B-vitamins below as well as a few extras thrown in for efficacy – you'll notice the benefits straight away! If you aren't supplementing with pills for your Vit-B needs, then just make sure to eat a diet rich in food sources for multiple different kinds of B-vitamins. Over time you will see gradual but tangible and strong effects.

Take a look at the list of the important B vitamins for your brain below:

Vitamin B12 (Cobalamin)

Cobalamin has been linked to heart and blood vessel problems, neurodegenerative disease, and Alzheimer's. Most cases of low levels of cobalamin are shown to be caused by problems in the gut that prevent the absorption of this naturally occurring B-vitamin through our diet.[14] We mentioned that increased homocysteine levels were linked with brain problems, well it turns out that they are also linked to the progression of dementia, AD, *as well as cobalamin deficiency.*[15]

I recommend taking B12, but specifically in the forms "Methylcobalamin" and "5-deoxyadenosylcobalamin" because these are the active forms and come with few to no adverse side effects in the body – they also work as opposed to doing nothing.[16] So, how do you get natural sources of these scarily named B-vitamins? Simple, natural food sources of this amazing vitamin include free-range fish wild-caught fish, poultry, eggs, and red meat. If you supplement try to get the scary-sounding named ones in addition to getting a good variety of these natural sources into your diet.[17]

Vitamin B6 (pyridoxal 5'-phosphate, known as "P5P")

Vitamin B6 in its active form (P5P) has been shown to enhance memory.[18] This vitamin is also responsible for regulating multiple metabolic processes linked to proteins – a link to Alzheimer's disease and memory performance for sure![19]

Vitamin B6 is utilized by the liver to help metabolize (break down, convert and store) glucose and it is required for liver and muscle cells to access energy stores of sugar to make glucose for use by the body – so it's important for weight loss in people with strong healthy livers. It's also used by the body to help make its own vitamin B3, serotonin, taurine, dopamine, norepinephrine, GABA, and histamine! (all very important compounds, many of which are important neurotransmitters!) Vitamin B6 is highly implicated in maintaining a stable nervous system.[20]

Vitamin B9 (Folate)

Having decreased numbers of vitamin B9 appears to be associated with chronic brain issues (e.g. Alzheimer's).[21] One study showed that folate deficiency reduced the ability of nerve cells to repair their genetic material – meaning that those cells became vulnerable to toxic exposure and death due to free radical damage. Folate has been proven to increase mental outcomes in many tests of cognitive performance.[22] [23]

What foods are rich in this awesome vitamin?

Organic cruciferous vegetables (dark leafy greens) have epic amounts of fabulous vitamin-B9.[24]

Vitamin B3 (Niacin)

Brain diseases like Alzheimer's are linked to deficiencies in Niacin.[25] Niacin also protects the heart and blood vessels from damage, and on top of that, niacin is a great antioxidant which is thought to be the main reason as to why it has all these beneficial effects.[26]

Where can I get dietary sources of niacin?

Find rich supplies of niacin in legumes and red meat. Your body can actually make this vitamin if it has sufficient amounts of P-5-P to work with as a building block, so that's another reason to take P-5-P in addition to the ones we already gave above!

Magnesium

Magnesium is one of the four most important supplements for healing your brain, boosting its performance, and maintaining its health once healthy. I keep mentioning Magnesium throughout the book and for very good reason – please take it for your brain!

Magnesium is a base metal element that is found in our bones, organs, and blood tissues.[27] It is a very important compound in our bodies. Magnesium, most of all, and in addition to all its other benefits and important functions, helps to protect and care for our mitochondria. Our mitochondria are like little biological power stations in the body. They are responsible for manufacturing, processing, and essentially creating energy in forms the body can use. Without our mitochondria working properly all our cells would die, we would have no energy to do anything, and our brains would be one of the first organs in the body to suffer as a result because our brains are so energy-hungry – they require a vast amount of our body's power output to handle everything that needs handling on a normal day-to-day basis.[28]

Ok, so the main thing you should think of when you hear the word 'Magnesium' is ENERGY and POWER for my BRAIN! What affects Magnesium levels in the body? Apart from eating enough food sources of magnesium, other things affect how much we can actually absorb from our gut, so gut health is important for our magnesium levels. Our kidneys affect our Magnesium levels as well as our levels of other micro minerals or metals like calcium, potassium, and sodium.

So, simply supplementing with Magnesium is not enough to ensure you have adequate amounts available inside the body for use. You need to look after your gut and make sure to have healthy kidneys, as well as make sure to get enough of all those other minerals I just mentioned. This basically means that if you want to supplement effectively with Magnesium you should really be taking a multi-mineral supplement. Not only is taking one pill for all your minerals easy and hassle-free, it actually makes the effects of each of the minerals stronger and more efficient – similar to the situation I described for the whole vitamin-B family of vitamins and supplementation.

Finally, but very importantly, it turns out that Magnesium is very important in the body for making proteins, protecting our delicate cell membranes from free radical damage, produce hormones, help muscles contract, aids our digestion and metabolism, *and helps neurons signal to each other!* These last points are what really propels Magnesium into superstar brain supplement status.[29]

Vinpocetine

Vinpocetine is a derivative of vincamine, a compound found inside the periwinkle plant. This extract proved very beneficial in improving cognitive function.[30] Vinpocetine has proven effective at improving cerebral blood flow in patients with dementia and AD. This suggests that it protects the nerves in your brain from damage.[31] [32] [33]

Vinpocetine improves cognition and memory in lab mice that had induced memory damage.[34] In patients with mild cognitive impairment, vinpocetine also improved cognition.[35]

OMEGA 3's - DHA (Docosahexaenoic Acid); EPA (Eicosapentaenoic Acid)

Both of these are long-chain essential dietary fatty acids that can be made inside the body from the breakdown of linoleic acid or found readily available in fish, walnuts, flax, and meat. The Inuit diet is incredibly high in these fats, their diets mostly containing frozen raw fish and blubber. Their population shows almost no cardiovascular problems, diabetes, arthritis, severe inflammatory conditions, or

Alzheimer's.[36] Both of these fatty acids are protective against metabolic inflammation. Inside the human body, DHA is found in the eyes, brain, and sperm cells.[37]

DHA is vital for maintaining ordinary brain function in adults and for brain growth in children.[38] Higher levels of dietary DHA have proven to increase learning ability and lower amounts will cause brain deficits.

DHA is one of the few fatty acids that are easily absorbable by the brain. A lack of DHA is also related to neurological deficits[39], depression, aggression, fibrosis, ADD, ADHD, alcohol fetal syndrome, alcoholism, inflammation, arthritis, pain, asthma, diabetes, a few cancers, and myocardial infarction. DHA reduces the proliferation of tumors and improves endothelial functioning.[40] It's very important to maintain proper levels of DHA in our diets, whether we have AD or not![41]

EPA is in the exact same boat as DHA, also having many of the same properties and found primarily in fish.[42] Both DHA and EPA aid in the metabolism 1of other lipids.

OMEGA 3's – ALA (Alpha Lipoic Acid)

Alpha-Lipoic Acid or just simply Lipoic Acid is an omega-3 fatty acid that is particularly good at fighting Alzheimer's disease as well as protecting and repairing brains.

Most of its benefits are because it is a potent anti-inflammatory and anti-oxidant, which helps protect nerve tissues from damage and degeneration.

So ALA is a 'protector' and it protects us from very reactive toxic chemical waste products that naturally form from the body's normal day-to-day processes. Not just that, but it performs the same function against environmental toxic exposure to pesticides, in addition to waste product build-up from poor or unhealthy dietary choices.

In addition to being a 'smart protector,' ALA is also very good at keeping our energy production processes in balance and regulating glucose metabolism. [43] [44] [45]

Amazingly, ALA is both water and fat-soluble, which means that it easily travels through all regions of the body – including the brain directly. In terms of direct brain results, ALA has been proven to prevent brain degeneration and deterioration, especially when its effects were combined with ALC (see above) – these two amazing 'smart compounds' seem to work best as a team.[46]

ALA alleviates symptoms linked to nerve damage and symptoms linked to nerve diseases and disorders in general, including the kinds of nerve damage we see in typically severe cases of diabetes.[47] [48] [49] It works as a major anti-inflammatory agent[50] and helps to guard against neurotoxicity, which would exacerbate the conditions of Alzheimer's,[51] Dementia, and Diabetic patients.

- Alpha-Lipoic Acid was shown to be effective at combating chemotherapeutically caused neuropathy.[52] [53] On the point of cancer and diabetes, Alpha-lipoic acid has been shown to majorly reduce toxicity in a patient with pancreatic cancer.[54] [55]
- Alpha Lipoic Acid aids energy production by allowing the body to produce cAMP, an energy building block to ATP.[56] [57]

Alpha-Lipoic Acid has been particularly in the spotlight for metal chelation, working very effectively with glutathione.[58] Mercury and Aluminum are some of the most toxic pollutants for your brain and are known factors in the development of Alzheimer's, Parkinson's, many other auto-immune diseases, as well as mitochondrial dysfunction-related disorders. [59]

In combination with other ingredients like vitamin E, C, and resveratrol, ALA successfully reduced the toxicity of insecticides in rats.[60] Alpha-lipoic Acid can also remove BPA (Bisphenol-A) from our bodies.[61] [62]

Other amazing finds on Alpha-Lipoic Acid Include:

- How it may effectively treat and prevents coronary heart disease.[63] [64] [65]
- May prove beneficial to Multiple Sclerosis patients in alleviating pain and inflammation.[66]
- Research has emerged showing that it may help remove, prevent, or reduce migraines.[67] [68]
- ALA may also be able to reduce the effects of HFCS-induced damage (lesions) on the pancreas[69] [70]

Vitamin C

Vitamin C is a powerful antioxidant compound and has for a long time been associated with immunity and health.[71] Vitamin C is required to regenerate oxidized Vitamin E. Berries and many orange fruits contain high doses of vitamin C.[72] Pretreatment with vitamin C reduced homocysteine levels (a sign of inflammation) which are correlated with vascular diseases when levels are high.[73] Generally speaking, 1g of vitamin C can be taken per day without safety issues provided that a suitably qualified health professional has evaluated any possible contra-indications.[74]

Vitamin E

Vitamin E is a vital nutrient for the body, just like Vitamin C. Make sure to find E vitamins in their natural and not synthetic form, gamma-tocopherol.[75] [76] Vitamin E has a large anti-inflammatory reach, being a potent antioxidant.[77] Vitamin E is required for cell signaling, particularly of inflammatory matters related to oxidative stress.[78]

Vitamin D3

Yes, the sunshine vitamin is great for brain health! Higher levels of vitamin D3 are associated with improved cognition in patients with degenerative brain disorders.[79] D3 has been shown to decrease the amount of amyloid-beta plaques in Alzheimer's patients,[80] as well as help repair the damage linked to these plaques.[81]

D3 is vital to the brain because it acts as a nerve cell protector and it brings calcium levels into balance in the body which is why it is commonly known to prevent rickets – calcium levels just so happen to be important for nerve cell activation too![82] Other important effects linked to D3 that many people don't commonly realize include:

- A deficiency of D3 is related to depression and reduced cognition in the elderly.[83]
- D3 deficiency is associated with all risk factors involved known for Alzheimer's disease.[84]
- Vitamin D3 taken with calcium has actually prevented hip and bone fractures in elderly women.[85]
- The anti-inflammatory properties of D3 help

important brain immune system cells to work properly (microglial cells).[86]

- D3 has the amazing ability to stimulate the growth of new nerve cells!!!![87]
- Many effects of vitamin D3 boost our immune systems positively.[88]

Vitamin D3 can be generated by getting enough sun exposure every day. However, as a supplement, it is quite easy to get, safe to use, and inexpensive. Supplementing with vitamin D3 makes sense if you live in a climate that has long hours without sun during cold winter months.

It also makes sense to supplement it if your body is already out of balance or you suffer from a disease/disorder, particularly one of the problems I described in chapter two of this book. In the latter case, since your body is already out of balance, you will probably need to take some strong measures upfront and supplement just until your body returns back to a form of basic functionality again – then make sure to get your sun, every single day.

Getting sun exposure is especially easy and fun to do if you combine it with an active hobby for exercise; good examples include hiking, active gardening, swimming, or surfing, but you can pretty much do your favorite thing outdoors in the sun (as long as it is active!) to get all the benefits. This means it is an absolute 'no-brainer', take vitamin-D3! Take it for your brain and the health of the rest of your body too.

Acetyl-L-Carnitine (ALC)

ALC is naturally produced in our bodies and is an essential amino acid building block.[89] Even since the preliminary studies done on ALC in the 90s, it has been noted that ALC improves symptoms of Dementia and Alzheimer's and slows the rate of brain deterioration.[90][91]

ALC reduces pain, reduces inflammation, and helps with certain symptoms linked to nerve damage in diabetes. One study even showed that ALC actually induced nerve regeneration.[92]

ALC has been well understood as a pain reliever, but as investigation dug deeper into this compound it was found that ALC actually works with neurotransmitters linked to acetylcholine, and we know from chapter one how important acetylcholine is for brain function.[93][94][95]

ALC has been shown to help with lots of different kinds of nerve-related toxic conditions (for example helping reduce nerve cell death when cancer patients have chemotherapy).[96] But, when combined with certain other compounds, it also can help our mitochondria out, as well as help to regulate blood sugar - this makes our brains happy because they don't get energy starved.[97]

Finally, if the above wasn't enough to convince you about the power of ALC for your brain, ALC was also shown to improve outcomes for symptoms of disorders like depression and Alzheimer's disease.[98]

The effects on depression and mood are particularly interesting for us since that is something many of you who are reading this might be struggling with, so the study that showed these benefits explained them by saying that ALC helps in different ways, here follows what they mentioned:

- AL-Carnitine is needed in the body for the metabolism of healthy fatty acids.
- ALC regulates brain energy levels as well as lipid metabolism in the brain. Lipids are required to protect all neurons and are concentrated in our brains.
- ALC also helps to regulate hormones that act on our nerves and other nerve acting biological compounds found naturally in the body.
- ALC is good at helping males retain their fertility because of some effects it has on sperm directly and beneficial effects on the heart and blood vessels indirectly.[99] [100]
- *ALC is necessary for healthy brain signaling, effective synapse communication, and for establishing neuron connections in the brain.*

Food Sources of Compounds for Brain Health

Extra Virgin Olive Oil

Olive Oil has been used in Mediterranean countries and some European countries for thousands of years. These countries which have olives and olive oil as a part of their heritage show significantly reduced numbers of Alzheimer's disease when compared to other countries.[101] [102]

Olive oil protects the brain from amyloid-beta plaques (ABP) by inhibiting their growth.[103] The phytochemical Oleocanthal is the culprit behind the amyloid-beta plaque inhibition, stimulating the release of enzymes that remove ABP shards out from the brain.[104] Other compounds in olive oil that protect against ABP's would be tyrosol and hydroxytyrosol.[105] Even in small doses, olive oil has been shown to remove many different types of beta plaques out of the brain.[106] Olive oil has been shown to improve memory and learning ability in mice.[107]

The anti-inflammatory properties of olive oil have been reviewed as being as effective as Ibuprofen.[108] There is also sufficient evidence to show that those who include pure olive oil in their diets have reduced risk and incidence of receiving cardiovascular problems[109] and coronary heart disease.[110]

Coconut Oil[111]

Natural health gurus have been preaching the word of coconut oil since research surfaced about it in the last decade or so. The coconut plant is one of the most sustainable plants on our planet, providing us with food, medicine, personal care, clothing, and building materials. Often thought of as a predominantly Indian or Indonesian plant, coconut varieties actually grow across every continent on the planet; barring Antarctica or permanently frosted over sections of Asia and North America. Cultures all around the globe have incorporated coconuts into their diet, from Brazil to Tanzania; New Guinea to Mexico.

Coconuts are one of the few plants that are capable of having over 100 benefits inside the human body alone. To begin with, coconut oil is full of medium-chain fatty acids[112] (MCF), which are easy to absorb by our bodies. MCF's get broken down into Ketones by our bodies and are an important secondary source of energy for our brains. Ketone research suggests ketones may be useful in ameliorating the effects of Alzheimer's disease. Beyond this, coconut oil itself has been shown to reduce the growth of amyloid-beta plaques by preventing them from aggregating – polyphenols and cytokines are responsible for this.

Coconut oil has been shown to have anti-diabetic properties and to help effectively combat cardiovascular diseases. Studies have linked coconut oil to be beneficial in the treatment of obesity, dyslipidemia, LDL cholesterol toxicity, high blood pressure, hypertension, insulin resistance, and glucose metabolism.[113] In a study done on rats, coconut oil was shown to have anti-inflammatory, analgesic (pain-alleviating), and antipyretic (fever breaking) effects.[114]

Berries!

Just about every single natural berry on our planet is rich in lipid-soluble antioxidant polyphenolic compounds. Some of these compounds include phenolic acids (like Ellagic acid, gallic acid, p-hydroxybenzoic acid, ferulic acid, and caffeic acid), and flavonoids (such as catechins, epicatechin, myricetin, quercetin, and kaempferol).[115]

The majority of the berries edible by humans can reduce inflammation and enhance energy production in the body. Berries are an important part of everyone's diet and should be included in any brain conscious person's shopping list.[116, 117]

Cranberries, blueberries, strawberries, chokeberries are rich sources of anthocyanins. These and anthocyanin extracts have shown the ability to aid in the metabolism of fats, reduce the aggregation of LDL cholesterol, improve glucose metabolism, and impart overall protection from the damage antioxidants do to our body. Anthocyanins have proven time and again to be able to enhance insulin sensitivity, promote the slow release of blood sugar, and effectively control the production of nitric oxide synthase, aiding all metabolic processes.[118]

As there are too many berries to cover, I am just going to focus on a few of the superstars for brain health.[119]

Pomegranate

Pomegranates have a long history of health and vitality linked to them. They have also been linked since ancient times with fertility, symbolizing the goddess in ancient traditions. With a treasure trove of abundant nutrients, energy-enhancing phytochemicals, and rich history in medicinal and culinary achievements, Pomegranate has got to be one of the healthiest foodstuffs on planet Earth.

The connection with pomegranates to the goddess oddly runs a bit deeper than one might think, as pomegranates contain one of the highest dietary sources of natural phytoestrogens. Improved blood flow, increased energy, and enhanced longevity have long been associated with this miraculous fruit. They have a gastronomical amount of antioxidant compounds and give our immune systems a boost with powerful protection against free radicals.[120]

One of the sugars inside pomegranate peels proved to self-destruct osteosarcoma cells by helping to stimulate the mitochondria.[121] These delicious berry fruits have also proven their 1aptitudes at preventing the formation of lung[122], breast[123], colon, and prostatic[124] cancers in the body.

Pomegranate improves mitochondrial functioning and radically reduces oxidative stress.[125] This red delicacy helps to reduce blood pressure, hypertension, and risk of cardiovascular disease, obesity, and type-2 diabetes.[126] Arterial plaques are encouraged to leave the body after pomegranate is ingested.[127] If you find an all-natural skincare product with pomegranate in it, you can now know that it repairs your skin, nourishes it, and has anti-aging properties.[128]

Pomegranate seed oil has liver-protecting properties in mice, suggesting it to be effective in treating fatty liver syndrome and liver-associated metabolic problems.[129] Pomegranate juice was shown to protect against radiation.[130] Pomegranate rinds have even been suggested as an effective treatment for AIDS.[131]

Strawberry

Strawberries, in general, have very high nutritional content, rich in polyphenols, phenolic acids, ascorbic acids, anthocyanins, ellagitannins, and antioxidant compounds. Studies have shown that the amount of these compounds vary across different varieties of strawberry.[132] It is noted that strawberries found in the Mediterranean diet are rich in these nutrients[133] and that the polyphenolic content of them reduces brain aging.[134] Wild strawberries contain the highest amounts[135] of the following health benefits:[136]

- Neuroprotection for the brain and against Alzheimer's neuropathy.[137] This is because of the antioxidant ability of strawberries phytochemicals to reduce oxidative stress-induced apoptosis in neuro-cells (PC12).[138]

- Ellagic Acid in strawberries prevents the growth of amyloid-beta plaques in the brain.[139]

- Unripe strawberries and blackberries have the highest ORAC values across berries that are still green.[140]

- Strawberry has proved to regulate LDL cholesterol formation[141] and after-meal blood lipid spikes by aiding in lipid metabolism in overweight people.[142] This suggests wild strawberries are a good addition to the diet of CVD patients or diabetics.

- Wild strawberries decrease CVD risk factors further; decreasing blood pressure, improving insulin sensitivity, and decreasing dyslipidemia.[143] Strawberries also reduce vascular adhesion, allowing the removal of atherosclerosis sites from the body.

- There is proof that strawberries act to remove

> blood clots and other arterial plaques as well as reduce the risk of heart attacks and strokes.[144]
>
> - Strawberries are also rich in vitamin C and E.[145]
> - In a study done on mice, wild strawberries that were grown via radiated conditions even proved effective at reducing memory deficits and enhancing brain cognition.[146]
> - Wild strawberries were shown to enhance the glycemic profiles of both white bread and rye bread by decreasing after-meal blood glucose spikes.[147]

Most commercial varieties have been genetically modified and shown to have increased sugar content, watering down the effects of these nutrients dramatically.[148] Eating phenolic-rich foods (like wild strawberries) with meals has been shown to reduce glucose-insulin-lipid surges in blood levels.[149]

Cranberry

Cranberries have been shown to reduce the levels of beta-amyloid plaques and toxicity caused by them.[150] Cranberries also have a high amount of resveratrol in them, which causes apoptosis in cancer cells as well as having antiproliferation properties (meaning that cancer spread and growth is inhibited).[151] Here we have a few more listed nutritional benefits of cranberries:

- Cranberry juice was found to decrease oxidized LDL levels and inflammation in metabolic syndrome patients. [152]
- Cranberries are excellent for working on problems in the kidneys or bladder. [153]
- It works to keep bacterial infections such as E.coli from attaching to the urinary tract walls. [154]
- It also imparts this to organisms in the gut and protects us from harmful intestinal pathogens. [155]
- Cranberries have been highlighted in the prevention of cancers. [156]
- Cranberries can help to treat ulcers when included in the diet.
- Cardiovascular patients will benefit from cranberries, as they restrict the accumulation of platelets or aggregations in the blood, reduce blood pressure, and decreases inflammation. [157]
- Cranberries have been suggested as an effective treatment against streptococcus mutans. [158]

Blueberry

Blueberries contain phenolic compounds Pterostilbene, Piceatannol, and resveratrol; all of which have abundant anticarcinogenic and antioxidant protecting effects in the body[159], especially the brain. These compounds help stimulate cognitive deficits associated with Alzheimer's and promote dopamine release by removing calcium deposits in the brain.[160]

This dark-colored berry protects the brain from degradation, decreased memory function, and reduced cognitive capacity, making it brilliant for use in the treatment of Alzheimer's disease.[161] Blueberry rich diets have shown a link to the growth of new nerve cells!

Blueberries lower all forms of blood pressure, decrease lipid oxidation, aggregation, and enhance insulin sensitivity.[162] They are rich in antioxidants, polyphenols, resveratrol, and omega-3 alpha-linolenic acid.[163]

A lot like blackberries and cranberries, blueberries cause apoptosis to occur in cancer cells and tumors. This is owing to the stilbene compound resveratrol, and Ellagic Acid found in many berries[164] (cranberries, blueberries, raspberries, strawberries, blackberries, and more).

High levels of quercetin were found in blueberries, bilberries, cranberries, lingonberries, gooseberries, and black or red currents.[165] Quercetin protects against oxidative damages against the DNA, particularly in lymphocytes.[166]

Raspberries

Raspberries have the highest ORAC values amongst many kinds of berries when ripe.[167] Jewel black raspberries have one of the highest antioxidant counts of all known natural berries.[168]

Raspberries have shown to have anti-proliferative (good against cancer) properties thanks to the high presence of Ellagitannins.[169]

Black raspberries inhibit the growth of esophageal tumors in lab rats.[170] Black raspberry was shown in the same experiment to inhibit proliferation, cause cancer cell apoptosis, as well as reducing inflammation. This is due to the ellagitannin content of raspberries.[171]

Raspberries are rich in vitamin C, anthocyanins, and Ellagitannins.[172] Raspberries also exhibit decreased vasodilation, suggesting it can help certain migraines and eye strain.

These delicious berries contain lymph-protective quercetin, alongside Ellagic acid and Ellagitannins.[173]

Commercial, store-bought, freshly picked GMO cultivars, and frozen raspberries all have similar polyphenolic and antioxidant content.[174] Wild raspberries have the highest amounts, though!

A study showed that Ellagitannins in raspberries are very easily absorbed by the stomach lining and no harmful by-products remain leftover.[175]

Cruciferous Vegetables

Cruciferous vegetables are supremely beneficial for the brain and help to maintain the health of your gut, internal organs, immune system, and prevent a whole host of problems linked to AD, MS, PD, and many other problems besides. Part of the reason cruciferous veggies are so good for the brain is that they tend to be very rich in many of the other compounds I describe elsewhere in this section – that makes them a great choice for your daily greens, in smoothies, salads, and main meals. Try to increase the amounts of these veggies you consume in your diet every day, and gradually they will become a great source of delicious brain-boosting support and protection.[176] [177]

Herbs, Spices, Nuts, & Other Sources of Potent Compounds for Your Brain

Rosemary

Throughout history, Rosemary has always been associated with remembrance, memory, and scholarship. Today this Mediterranean plant is a common household plant and it's cultivated throughout all warmer regions of the planet. Rosemary has been used traditionally to enhance memory and focus[178], reduce gut contractions, provide respiratory relief, and soften hair. Rosemary has been shown to exhibit all these effects, as well as liver protection, cancer prevention, and digestion improvement.[179]

Carnosic acid is essential for Alzheimer's disease treatment and prevention, reducing beta-amyloid toxicity.[180] In an experiment carried out on components of Rosemary, it was discovered that Rosemary has an almost aggressive free radical binding ability and has effective antimicrobial properties. Rosemary can reduce numbers of both gram-positive and gram-negative bacteria, even killing off yeasts. The phenolic compounds responsible for this inside Rosemary are carnosic acid, carnosol, and rosmarinic acid (a derivative of caffeic acid).[181]

Another study done on the same above compounds (carnosic acid, carnosol, and rosmarinic acid) in rosemary and oregano showed that oregano has higher amounts of these three compounds. Both Rosemary and Oregano were shown to have high antioxidant capacity.[182]

Carnosic acid, along with the phenolic diterpenoids: rosmanol, carnosol, and epirosmanol, conferred mitochondrial protection against oxidative stress. In the same study, carnosic acid alone protected blood cells from free radical damage.[183]

Rosemary has been shown to enhance cognitive function and uplift moods.[184] A study done revealed that Rosemary acts as an anti-depressant, regulating Dopamine, serotonin, and GABA pathways in the brain. Rosemary also regulated the neurotransmitters norepinephrine, serotonin, acetylcholine, and dopamine.[185] All of these pathways and neuro-transmitters are required to build chemicals that regulate positive moods, good sleep, digestion, and brain health. Further research shows that the powerful antioxidant effects of rosemary polyphenols protect the cell lines in these pathways.[186] Rosemary acts similarly to Prozac (fluoxetine), except that unlike Prozac, Rosemary does not have any undesirable side effects that detract from learning capacity.[187]

Rosemary is beneficial in the treatment of cancer, Alzheimer's disease, cataracts, ischemic heart disease, atherosclerosis, disease-related inflammation, liver toxicity, asthma, metabolic disorders, diabetes[188], and digestive problems. A 2012 study showed Rosemary to have analgesic (pain killer) properties.[189]

Rosemary has been shown to reduce blood cholesterol in rats.[190] Another study indicated that rosemary reduces blood sugar levels and improves lipid metabolism.[191]

Rosemary and Sage both destroy tumors[192] as well as inhibit lipid peroxidation.[193] The same study reveals Rosemary to have antifungal and antibacterial properties, protecting against E.coli, Salmonella, candida, and more. Rosemary effectively treated Streptococcus in fish.[194]

Lemon Balm

Lemon Balm contains many beneficial polyphenolic antioxidants, including hydroxycinnamic acid, gallic acid, caffeic acid and derivatives, rosmarinic acid, naringenin, naringin, and hesperidin.[195] Lemon balm extract was shown to have high amounts of phenols, phenolic acids, proanthocyanins, flavonoids, gamma-tocopherol (Vitamin E), and vitamin C.[196]

Lemon Balm has a history of being able to aid in the treatment of spasms, as well as being anti-bacterial and alleviating anxiety.[197] This botanical also has a history of treating Alzheimer's and dementia patients, allowing them to hold their focus for extended periods.[198] In a 2004 study done, lemon balm was shown to improve cognitive speed, increase self-rated calmness levels and reduce stress and alertness.[199]

Mellissa Officinalis has been shown to regulate our moods and enhance cognitive performance further by acting upon our central nervous system. Lemon balm can bind to nicotinic and muscarinic receptors (neuron cells that form part of the acetylcholine neurotransmitter).[200] Lemon balm has been shown to inhibit pain by binding to these receptors and also works on the L-arginine-nitric oxide pathway.[201] Sage and rosemary share these same properties with lemon balm[202] and are all indicated in the treatment of Alzheimer's disease. Early studies have shown that Parkinson's and

Alzheimer's both exhibit symptoms of low levels of dopamine and acetylcholine neurotransmitters.[203]

Lemon Balm decreases anxiety and works as an anti-depressant in rats.[204] In a study done, lemon balm was shown to reduce stress levels and increase GABA levels in mice.[205]

Anti-diabetic properties have been spotted in lemon balm, which exhibited the ability to prevent the growth of Glycation End Products.[206] This suggests Lemon Balm is good to include in the diets of people with diabetes, cardiovascular disease, Alzheimer's, cancer, metabolic conditions, and neurodegenerative disorders.

Lemon balm is shown to bind to iron and free radicals in the body, which pulls the iron out of the system.[207] In the same experiment, lemon balm extract was proven to reduce cyto-toxicity and reduce DNA damage by preventing deoxyribose deterioration. On this same note, another study confirmed further DNA protection against the effects of radiation when lemon balm was included in the diets of radiology staff.[208] Lemon balm has also been proven effective at treating Herpes Simplex virus type 2[209]

Thyme

Thymus Vulgaris, known commonly as Thyme, has been used globally for centuries in many continental traditional medicine remedies. Thyme has a reputation for alleviating coughs, spasms, and inflammation. This herb is also a powerful antioxidant and antimicrobial. Thymol is used in antiseptic mouthwashes and has plaque destructive characteristics.

Thyme has been approved by the German Commission Expert Panel for use in the treatment of respiratory inflammation, whooping coughs, and bronchitis. Thymol has antifungal properties too and has been used to disinfect skin wounds.[210] Important aging-related biomarkers improved in the brain of rat fed with thymol extract.[211] Thyme consists of 49% Thymol and was found to maintain higher levels of polyunsaturated fatty acids in the brains, hearts, kidneys, and livers of mice.[212]

Thyme extract was shown to lower cholesterol and fat as well as improve liver health in chickens.[213] Like rosemary, sage, and mint, thyme has a high concentration of rosmarinic acid, as well as smaller amounts of caffeic acid, gallic acid, vanillin, and more.[214] Rosmarinic acid has proven to prevent amyloid-beta plaque formation.[215] Further research has shown rosmarinic acid to reduce the aggregation of blood lipids, as well as improve the activity of the acetylcholine neurotransmitter.[216]

Approximately 90% of thyme sourced polyphenols can be extracted into olive oil to enhance the oil.[217] Thyme is abundant in salicylic acid[218], the main active principle in aspirin imbuing it with its painkilling effects and ability to reduce fevers.

When thyme was combined with ginger in a tea infusion, they showed to have combined potent antioxidant ability and were recommended for use to decrease alcohol toxicity.[219]

Thyme has proven that it can remove the parasite Toxocara canis from rat brains as well as protect the brain from larvae damages.[220]

One study showed that a spray containing 2% of alpha-terpinene, found in thyme, can even act as an alternate mosquito repellent.[221]

Thyme contains luteolin and apigenin, sharing in many of the same properties as olives.[222] The research confirmed that thyme and marjoram both have protective antioxidant and toxicity lowering effects[223] A few species of thyme has been shown to protect[224] against oxidative damage done to DNA in lymphocyte tissue.[225]

A study done revealed that thyme was effective at removing cadmium chloride from the body, further confirming that cadmium chloride creates severe brain damage over time.[226]

Thyme has been suggested in the treatment of multiple scle-rosis[227] due to its powerful array of flavonoids.[228] Thyme has been shown to modulate the thyroid gland and provide liver-protective properties.[229] Thyme honey has been shown to have enhanced antimicrobial and antifungal characteristics thanks to the compounds bees collect in thyme flower pollen.[230] The same honey in a separate study revealed to abolish breast, endometrial, and prostate cancers.[231] Thyme has been implicated in the prevention of cancers along with many other similar herbs in other studies done.[232]

An analysis of thyme and marjoram revealed that the polyphenolic content of each went as high as 84mg per 1g of the herb![233]

Cinnamon

Cinnamon is rich in two powerful brain-boosting compounds; cinnamaldehyde and epicatechin, which both decrease levels of tau protein in the brain.[234] Tau is implicated in Alzheimer's disease because it aggregates (clumps) in the brain, which causes damage to the brain over time. In terms of AD, one of the main research findings that support its benefits for this particular disease is that it has potent blood-glucose-lowering effects (reductions of up to 29% were recorded in one study).[235]

Cinnamaldehyde has been shown to reduce oxidative byproducts like acrolein. In the same study, Epicatechin was shown to especially protect tau from abnormal mutations.[236] By decreasing the amount of glycation end products in the brain, these two compounds help micro-tubules to function properly and prevent neurofibrillary tangles. Cinnamon was proven to reduce amyloid-beta plaque formation in mice models.[237]

Cinnamon has been indicated in the prevention of diabetes type 2, metabolic syndrome, and cardiovascular diseases. Cinnamon was shown to aid all of these by reducing inflam-mation, weight gain, glucose-lipid blood levels, improving mitochondrial functioning, insulin resistance[238], glycation end products as well as glycation formation.[239] Cinnamon's superior antioxidant ability allows it to retrieve reactive carbonyls, reducing the formation of glycation.[240] Cinnamon managed to protect pancreatic beta cells from oxidative damage, aiding digestion, and upregulating insulin secretion.[241] Little known to many people, Cinnamon also kills of helicobacter pylori, making it a potentially effective part of an anti-ulcer treatment protocol.[242]

The polyphenols inside cinnamon reduce swelling in nerve cells as well as improve their energy production.[243] [244] Cinnamaldehyde is currently considered to be the main compound in cinnamon that is responsible for preventing inflammation of nerve cells and thus by extension protecting nerve cells from damage linked to that inflammation.[245]

One study showed that an extract from cinnamon caused apoptosis in cervical cancer cells.[246] Cinnamon is shown to promote the production of Brain-Derived Neurotrophic Factor, which encourages the growth of neuronal cells.[247] This was also suggested as an effective treatment for Parkinson's disease, as well as Alzheimer's disease.

The aqueous cinnamon extract was further shown to protect against oxidative damages caused by BPA (Bisphenol-A) and octylphenol, both of which are not healthy. The study went on to show that cinnamon protects against damages to the kidneys, testicles, and brains.[248] Cinnamon enhanced the activity of malfunctioning lead acetate-induced sperm cells in rats.[249] Cinnamon achieved this by protecting against the damaging effects of lead acetate.

Cinnamon protected Prostaglandin E2 (PGE2) production, which mediates vasodilation, anti-inflammatory responses, and sleep regulation. Cinnamon will help to improve sleep in patients who suffer from insomnia.[250]

Resveratrol

Resveratrol is a polyphenol that is an essential part of everyone's diets, aiding the body with a large number of processes. It is found in Pomegranates, boiled peanuts, and red grape skins, dark chocolate, and red wine.[251]

In regards to Alzheimer's, multiple studies have shown resveratrol to be strongly neuroprotective[252] because it reduces amyloid-beta plaque growth and formation as well as acting as a strong antioxidant.[253] Resveratrol increases levels of SIRT1 protein, which protects the brain's neurons from deterioration and toxicity.[254]

Derivatives of Resveratrol are known as stilbenoids or stilbenes. These are proving to be equally as desirable as resveratrol.[255] Pterostilbene is a stilbene that has a very similar profile to resveratrol, having anti-inflammatory benefits that combat brain aging and help to reduce amyloid-beta build-up in the brain.[256]

Ashwagandha

"Withania Somnifera," or, "Indian Ginseng," are two alternative names for Ashwagandha, a plant native to India. Indian Ginseng looks to be a very promising treatment for Alzheimer's, Parkinson's, spinal cord injury[257] , and neurological disorders[258], commonly used in Ayurvedic practice to enhance cognition.[259]

Ashwagandha root extract has revealed to scientists in a study that it promotes the growth of dendrites and axons when looking at increased mRNA markers.[260] Dendrites in subjects were shown to have extended in length, meaning this plant literally rebuilds back your brain!

Ashwagandha has been shown to prevent copper-induced oxidative lipid aggregation as well as provide antioxidant neuronal protection to spinal cords in the elderly.[261] The antioxidant properties of this plant extend to being an anti-stress adaptogen, proving effective at reducing stress in rats.[262] [263] This adaptogenic property of Indian Ginseng to reduce stress improves all functions of the body, including reduced blood-glucose levels, reduced blood plasma levels, decreased blood pressure, improved cognition, improved immune function, and reduced physical depression.[264]

Two amazing compounds found in this plant include two triterpenoids, withanolide A, and withaferin A. Both of these can destroy tumors as well as anti-angiogenic characteristics[265] (it prevents tumors from growing blood vessels). This plant also was shown to have anti-cancerous properties when had in a tea.[266]

Ashwagandha has anti-inflammatory effects, hematopoietic characteristics, and also improves the functioning of the immune system.[267] Ashwagandha protects the endocrine system, cardiovascular system, and the central nervous system. This plant prevents the accumulation of amyloid-beta plaques in the brain of Alzheimer's-induced mice.[268] [269] Studies suggest that this plant could be a potent anti-depressant; working on the acetylcholine neurotransmitter pathway[270], repairing DNA damages, and reducing the effects of toxicity in neurons and glioma cells.[271]

However, these two compounds are not the only ones that work inside this amazing plant. In an experiment done, scientists managed to isolate an additional 4 compounds that have much the same effects.[272] Indian Ginseng is full of catechins, which are potent antioxidant polyphenolic compounds.[273]

Ashwagandha has been shown to improve mitochondrial functioning as well as arthritis and memory loss.[274] Another study mentions that Ashwagandha can combat infection indirectly by enhancing the microbial killing potential of our immune response as well as having antimicrobial properties itself.[275] Indian ginseng is also notably fantastic for use in anti-aging protocols, and for improving respiratory and cardiovascular health.

Walnuts

Walnuts along with berries are associated with longevity[276] and protecting against neurodegeneration.[277] [278] Walnuts prevent the aggregation of proteins in the brain.[279] Walnuts further protect the brains of Alzheimer's patients by preventing amyloid-beta plaque cytotoxicity.[280] In the same study, walnuts proved effective at protecting DNA damages. Walnuts have been linked to improved cognition and decreased memory deficit in mice with Alzheimer's.[281] Walnut extract destroys neurofibrillary tangles in the brain and prevents them from forming.[282]

The decent concentration of omega-3 fatty acids is suggested to play a very supportive role in the prevention of Alzheimer's disease.[283] Omega-3's[284] ameliorate blood clotting, hormones, digestion, muscle contraction, and the movement of nutrients into cells. Walnut extract is shown to reduce symptoms of vascular dementia, as well as improve cardiovascular health.[285] These fatty acids in walnuts also protect the brain from inflammation in the hippocampus, indirectly improving cognition and memory.[286]

Walnuts chelate iron, remove many free radical particles from the body, and improve activity in the acetylcholine neurotransmitter.[287]

The Four 'Best' Supplements for Your Brain Health

This Chapter has explored so many supplements, foods, fruits, nuts, herbs, teas, and extracts from plants that can help your brain that it is difficult to know which ones you should focus on. Although this list is of potent tools is an incredible resource for you to draw from as you explore your preferred way to support your brain, it's useful to point out a few of the 'superstars' from that list here just to empha-size the safest and most efficient options.

Overall, four supplements keep cropping up as being extremely powerful in terms of healing the brain, maintaining the brain's current health, and supporting and improving a healthy brain's functioning. So in that spirit, the four most beneficial supplements that you should be taking are mentioned below.

Omega-3's (Omega-3 Fatty Acids)

These are so beneficial for so many factors that support healthy brains and healthy bodies that every plan to support the brain should include them. For a comprehensive description of their benefits for you please refer to the appropriate section in this chapter. These fatty acids are greatly needed for the health of your body and your brain. Taking them regularly will, in the long run, have massive benefits for your heart, blood vessels, and brain.

Vitamin D (particularly Vitamin D3)

Many people work indoors, avoid sun exposure, and use strong sunscreen. This helps to avoid overexposure to harmful ultraviolet radiation, reduce skin cancer risks, and prevent sunburn and premature aging. The downside is that many people nowadays are pretty deficient in this important vitamin. If you want to see how important vitamin D3 is for your body and brain please refer back to the vitamin D3 discussion earlier in this chapter. It is possible to get your quota of D3 by making sure you get enough sun exposure every day. But some countries may not have sufficient sunny weather all year round, and many aspects of the modern western diet put pressure on our bodies to use up this important vitamin. Supplementing with vitamin D3 has so many benefits for the body and brain it would be criminal not to take it regularly an hour before sleep.

Vitamin B (The whole family of B-Vitamins)

In part II of this book, I mentioned that many of the B-vitamins have potent brain protecting and boosting properties. The other factor to consider with B-vitamins is that they work better when you take them together. So, the easiest way to powerfully boost your brain support is to simply take a vitamin-B 'complex' supplement. A vitamin-B 'complex' is just a collection of many different B-vitamins all put into one tablet or supplement. Taking them all together is the best way to maximize their benefits – doing it this way also makes it easier for you to take them since you only need one tablet to get the benefits of many vitamins.

That being said, the main B-vitamin that is known to be super healthy for the brain is vitamin-B12. But there are also plenty of other B-vitamins that are also very important for our brains too. The B-vitamins are important for reducing stress, protecting blood vessels, promoting blood cell production, and generally keeping the heart, blood vessels, and brain in good shape as a unit. Make sure that your B-complex has sufficient amounts of B12 for optimal brain health and performance.

Magnesium

I talked at length about the impressive benefits of magnesium for the brain and body. To be honest, no brain-boosting plan will be effective without it. Make sure you include this one in your supplement list. Better yet, why not take a 'multi-mineral' supplement daily that has a good amount of magnesium in it along with many other important minerals and micronutrients – this would be the most efficient, minimum effort way to benefit. A multi-mineral supplement will be beneficial for multiple body systems and organs. Magnesium is particularly good for preventing migraines, and supporting the heart and blood vessels – it also supports individual cells' daily functioning.

III

BRINGING IT ALL TOGETHER

WHAT TO INCREASE/DECREASE | SUPPLEMENTATION GUIDE | SMOOTHIES | PRACTICAL TIPS & ADVICE

9

A PRACTICAL PLAN OF ACTION

We know from Chapter 1 that there are critical systems and factors that your brain relies on to be healthy and perform optimally. We also know from discussions all throughout the book so far that there are powerful tools that you can use to support each of these factors. Not only are there tools like supplements and potent bioactive compounds that boost the health of your body systems to support your brain, but there are also behavioral strategies that influence your brain too.

These behavioral strategies are things like making sure you sleep deeply and regularly; making sure to reduce your stress and anxiety; making sure to exercise body and mind; and consistently choosing to live day-by-day to support your brain health and overall health.

Speaking more specifically, a practical plan of action that will boost your brain's performance and health should incorporate everything at your disposal to tackle each key factor of brain performance simultaneously. This means that we can list the different strategies you should be engaging with clearly. Take a look at the list below:

- Eat right for your gut microbiome and support your gut-brain axis
- Take powerful beneficial supplements
- Be mindful of your immediate environment at home, work, and inside your body
- Reduce stress
- Sleep properly
- Exercise
- Tackle any chronic illness (e.g. Alzheimer's disease) or neurological problem (e.g. migraines, or chronic pain) that you may currently be facing have with the methods presented in chapters 3 and 4

The above list is an example of all the things you should be doing simultaneously to heal your brain, support your body health, and combat depression, anxiety, and stress. The best results will come from a comprehensive approach that tackles your brain health at every single level at the same time.

Each point above synergizes with other points on the list. For example:

Exercise reduces stress which leads to better sleep leading to better nutrition more energy and healthier bodies clearer thinking and optimized choices which leads to better management of your daily stresses and obligations which creates more harmony in your environment which reduces your exposure to toxic factors in your environment which leads to less chronic pain and inflammation making it more likely that you will exercise feeding back into reducing your stress and so on.

Hopefully, you can see that once you get these factors working in your favor, they feedback in a positive loop of ever-increasing wellness that gradually raises your health status to an optimal equilibrium point. Supplementation is helpful in the beginning to kick start those systems in your body that are so far out of balance already that they do not respond well to behavioral changes on their own.

Eventually, the hope is that your life changes so radically that supplementation won't be necessary on daily basis - just useful from time to time over periods of extreme stress or seasonal illness to bolster your status over troubling times.

Finally, behavioral changes are difficult to stick with, unless you see the results for yourself and feel the benefits – that is why journaling your day-to-day experience, or having a friend witness your progress and mirror it back to you with encouragement and feedback can be an important way for you to measure your success and keep motivated. Ultimately the changes you make today will become habits that you do not even think about anymore – it will just be the way you live your life - your 'natural groove'.

So, in the remainder of this chapter, I want to point out the practical implementation of the theory I have presented in this book so far. Let's start with a general remark about the aims of your choices and then move on to concrete examples of what to do after that.

Primary Aim: Reclaim Your Brain by Preventing & Repairing Damage in your brain and gut tissues

We want to remove all the causes that result in neuro-oxidative damage. So anything you do for your brain must ultimately halt and repair damage to your nerves and support their functioning.

The Practical Approach to reclaiming your brain aims to create the following results for you:

- Optimizing energy production, help to regulate blood glucose levels naturally.

- Reducing or eliminating inflammation (particularly in the brain tissues and gut)
- Eliminate sources of toxicity and remove accumulated toxins.
- Boost your immune function.
- Correct any nutritional deficiencies.
- Bring your gut into balance via good dietary changes
- Bring your moods into balance as an intentional side effect of repairing gut and brain health.
- Support the heart and blood vessels.

How do you do this? The rest of this chapter makes suggestions based on what we have discussed so far in this book.

Exercise

Based on our discussion of exercise in this book the best approach would be to try to do 30 minutes of moderate exercise 3-5 days per week. This applies to cardiovascular exercise. It is important to start gently and appropriately depending on your current level of fitness and state of health. The suggestion is the ideal you should work towards, but you may not be in a position to handle moderate-intensity exercise straight away. Work with a professional to evaluate your health and fitness status, come up with a plan that leads to moderate exercise 3 to 5 times a week for 30 minutes.

Don't forget that hobbies can also involve exercise if they are active. An added bonus is getting good sun exposure if your activity is outdoors. Exercise is great if it has a low impact on the joints, so things like hiking, long walks, swimming, cycling, and anything in a similar vein would be perfect ways to get your moderate weekly exercise without damaging your body.

Reduce Stress & Sleep Properly

Take a look at the chapter on stress and exercise earlier on in this book. What I recommend is that you can use any strategy from there that makes sense to you. Meditation is a great activity with proven brain-enhancing effects as well as stress-reducing side effects.

Exercise reduces stress too, and, of course, makes it easier to get to sleep, sleep longer, and have a better quality of sleep when you do get it.

Speaking of sleeping properly, the best sleep practices supported in the scientific literature is to get to sleep at nearly the same time every day and not to sleep too long or too little. You only need between 7 and 8 hours of sleep per night, not more, and not less than that. So the ideal range is probably seven and a half hours per night. Avoid stimulants like coffee or caffeine, or other similar things after 4pm in the afternoon. Try to keep naps to a minimum, but if you do nap make it no longer than 30 minutes. Try to only enter your bed when you are about to sleep, reduce the wakeful activities you might be doing while you are in bed so that your body learns that being in bed is linked to 'sleep time'.

The above sleep advice is linked to something called "sleep hygiene" and they are great ways to ensure you aren't hyper-activated (in terms of your brain activity) when it comes to sleeping time. If you simply cannot fall asleep then avoid pharmaceutical sleeping pills which have nasty side effects and are known to be extremely addictive (as in the case of barbiturates). A simple natural solution that can easily replace sleeping drugs is Melatonin which is very safe to use, well-tolerated, is a potent antioxidant, and has been prescribed for years to help people with jet lag. Melatonin is also naturally produced in the body, so taking about 1mg an hour before you want to go to sleep for five nights a week should work wonders. The remaining two nights a week it is best to give your body a chance to handle your natural mela-tonin secretion on its own to mitigate any 'downregulation' – a state where the body slightly decreases its own produc-tion of melatonin because it is getting so much from external sources.

Work with your favorite health professional to use melatonin properly.

If you exercise, and you sleep properly, you will reduce your stress levels, which make it much easier to sleep properly and exercise - A great positive health cycle that you should try to set up to work for you.

What Kind of Food?

This one is really simple, just follow a Mediterranean diet. Lots of olive oil, olives, avocadoes, light meat portions of lamb, free-range ethically raised chicken, and so on. I have provided a lot of discussion of diet and eating for your gut microbiome. If you get your food right, the little organisms in your gut will be happy, which will affect every aspect of your health including your moods, motivation, drive, the efficiency of absorption, and of course, your brain.

Nevertheless, there are some concrete tips I can give you to put the theory of the book into practice effectively. Consider the following general and specific tips and advice as a great start to shifting away from your current eating style towards something that enhances your brain. After these general tips and suggestions I give you two example smoothie recipes that are packed full of brain-enhancing health-boosting ingredients (easy and delicious too); consider daily smoothies as a form of nutritional medicine for your gut, body, and brain – they are your daily 'aces in the hole' and you should be making use of them or something like them to accelerate your health.

Changing your diet and your preferences is not an easy task. Start gradually by implementing the tips you think you can do. Then over time keep adding one more change until you have it all changed in your favor. One tip worth its weight in gold in terms of changing your cooking and eating preferences is to look at your current set of favorite recipes and substitute the unhealthy ingredients for similar ingredients that are actually healthy. For example, instead of using margarine, or butter, try substituting unflavored coconut oil or olive oil. Instead of sugar, perhaps add fruit to your meal, or a healthy substitute like stevia root powder, or honey. Substitutions tend to keep your favorite recipes intact, tasting the same or similar, but radically increase their health status and nutritional value whilst preventing inflammation and toxic byproducts.

The tips, advice, smoothies, and supplementation suggestions follow… enjoy!

GENERAL THINGS YOU SHOULD DO...

What to Increase

- Apples, Pomegranate (May use 100% pure unsweetened juice)
- Blueberries, Cranberries, Raspberries, Red Grapes & Blackcurrants
- Olive oil
- Coconut oil/milk/water
- Fish and marine oils from uncontaminated oceans
- Nuts & seeds – especially walnuts
- Cruciferous vegetables
- Legumes
- Onions & Garlic
- Cinnamon
- Cocoa – 1 block dark chocolate or warm drink
- Ground black pepper
- Saffron, Rosemary, Thyme, Turmeric, and curcumin
- Lemon Balm
- Cocoa – Dark chocolate (in wise moderation)
- Himalayan salt
- Green Tea – drink 3 to 5 cups daily but not after 4pm (the caffeine found naturally in green tea can keep you awake)
- Filtered water – drink 4 to 6 liters daily with a squeeze of lemon – an especially good first drink of the day to get the bile juices flowing and kick start your metabolism.

General Dietary Guidelines that are Beneficial

- Low Glycemic Index Fruit and Vegetables
- Increase dietary intake of Polyphenolic / Antioxidant foods
- Increase alkaline food
- Complex carbohydrates – whole foods and grains
- Foods with high fiber content
- Foods high in B Vitamins
- Foods rich in omega-3's (ALA/DHA/EPA) and the ONLY healthy omega-6 (GLA)
- Organic non-genetically modified foods
- Introduce more raw foods into your diet through potent smoothies
- A daily brain-boosting smoothie of your choice

What to avoid

- Foods with High Glycemic Index
- Eliminate all simple sugars in your diet
- Artificial sweeteners especially- Aspartame & HFCS
- Additives, food colorants, heavy metals, pesticides
- Plastic in containers & lining food packaging - BPA
- Refined and processed foods including commercially refined salt

- Smoked foods – nitrosamines in cold-smoked luncheon meats
- Fruit juice – fructose
- Alcohol & smoking & Television
- Unhealthy fats – Hydrogenated, tans-fatty acids & saturated fats
- Dairy products – casein, butter, cream
- Wheat, pastries & pasta – gluten, gliadin
- White refined rice
- Avoid animal fats - Limit red meat intake to wild game in moderation
- Genetically Modified Foods and inorganic farming practices
- Microwaved foods
- Grain-fed livestock (avoid all of them)

Beneficial lifestyle Factors

- Physical exercise is essential – 20 to 30 minutes per day low impact
- Deep regenerative sleep – refer to Foods to Aid Sleep
- Meditation Exercises – mindfulness and stress relaxation
- Learn something new daily – especially a musical instrument or singing

- Mental stimulation through activities such as crosswords, scrabble, Sudoku, puzzles, bridge, and chess, learning something new like a language or some other mental skill
- Swimming, hiking, hobbies, strong social connections (Socialize with friends)
- Raw organic smoothies that are packed with natural digestive enzymes

The Four Basic Supplements You Should Take

The following four supplements are the easiest and most potent for you to take to get the maximum benefit with a minimum of fuss.

- Omega-3's (Omega-3 Fatty Acids)
- Vitamin D (particularly Vitamin D3)
- Vitamin B (The whole family of B-Vitamins)
- Magnesium

For a more detailed description of their amazing benefits and properties definitely revisit the appropriate sections in Chapter 8.

However, if you would like to get the maximum benefit that you can from all the information in chapter 8 of this book, then consider following the advanced supplementation program that I present next.

General advice and dosage for taking the above four supplements are included in the advanced table below and elsewhere in the book for your convenience.

Please bear in mind that natural supplements are extremely powerful healing tools and they should be taken under supervision with the utmost care and respect to ensure your safety, health, and happiness.

An Advanced Supplementation Protocol for a High Functioning Healthy Brain

On the next page, you will find a table listing every single one of the most potent natural supplements that can help to heal your brain, boost it, or maintain it in optimal condition. The table is just a guide or skeleton and indicates the effective dosages for someone who is looking to take radical action to heal and improve their brain should they be suffering from a degenerative disorder like Alzheimer's or Parkinson's disease. The table indicates when supplements are best taken in the day, an effective, tolerable dose from the research literature, and the name of each compound. This is only a rough guide, and it should only be used under supervision.

One of the best uses of the table that follows is a reference or a convenient summary of the most beneficial and important supplements that you could ever hope to make use of for your brain. I have already recommended the four best supplements for you to use because just by using those four together with good eating, exercise, and stress reduction, those four supplements will do 80% of the heavy lifting. If you want to do the 100% optimal plan, consider making use of the advanced supplementation protocol as a start – take it to your doctor and begin there, adding and subtracting items from it as best fits your unique profile. The advanced protocol is meant to be a skeleton for you to work with an experienced suitably qualified professional – it is powerful and brings the final 20% benefit into the picture.

Supplement	Breakfast		Lunch		Dinner		Dose
	Before	After	Before	After	Before	After	
Daily Brain Booster Smoothie	X		X		X		Between meals
Carnitine (L-Acetyl Carnitine)		X		X		X	450 mg
Vitamin E (Gamma tocopherol = 200 μg)		X					350 - 400 mg
Methylcobalamin (sub-lingual)	X				X		800 - 1000 mcg
Alpha-Lipoic Acid (ALA) – R Form		X		X		X	150 - 200 mg
Resveratrol		X		X			450 - 500 mg
Phosphatidylserine		X		X		X	80 - 100 mg
Flaxseed Oil (cold-pressed organic)		X					½ to 1 Tablespoon
Grape Seed Extract		X		X		X	25 - 50 mg
Vitamin D3						X	650 - 800 IU
Magnesium						X	500 mg
Vitamin C	X		X		X		500 mg
Melatonin						X	1-2 mg, abstain for 2 evenings per week Dosages of between 9-15 mg can be tolerated easily 9 – 15 mg
Multi-vitamin (B3 / B6 / Folate must be included)		X					Follow package insert
Multi-mineral (Chromium /Zinc/ Magnesium included)						X	Follow package insert
Ginkgo biloba		X		X		X	70 mg

Note: It is important to let your health practitioner know that you intend to follow this protocol. Under no circumstances should you stop a prescribed medical protocol without consulting your doctor first. This supplemental program is a guideline only and cannot be taken without first consulting a medical expert.

Smoothies to Use, Smoothies to Choose

Making and drinking smoothies is one of the easiest and most delicious ways to benefit from the information in this book. For a bit of variety, I have suggested two slightly different smoothies. Each recipe is great for your brain, but each is also really good for something else too. I want to encourage you to use these recipes as examples for you to take inspiration from and create your own concoctions that you love. Choose your ingredients from the powerful foods and tools that I introduced to you in Part II of this book. Look for food sources of magnesium, or omega-3's, or target some of your favorite fruits and berries – the sky is the limit, and your brain will thank you, along with your tongue too, enjoy!

DAILY SMOOTHIE 01 – "THE DAILY BRAIN BOOSTER"

The easiest and most delicious way to heal, maintain and boost brain performance

This smoothie is your 'all-purpose, general brain health smoothie. It is potent, helpful, tasty, and the things in it come from the researched sources in this book. It is particularly good for people with Alzheimer's disease, but it will benefit anyone who has it ever single day. Feel free to vary your smoothies from time to time if you want a little variety.

Ingredients

1 cup of coconut milk

1 cup mango pieces

1 banana

1 tablespoon coconut oil

1 heaped teaspoon turmeric powder or freshly grated turmeric

1 teaspoon moringa powder

½ teaspoon cinnamon

½ teaspoon ginger

A pinch of Himalayan salt

2 tablespoons chia seeds

1 tablespoon flaxseed oil (cold-pressed)

½ cup washed organic blueberries or berry of your choice

1 tablespoon of Maca

1 slice of pineapple

(½ teaspoon black ground pepper – optional, helps bioavailability, choose on taste preference)

Method

Blend all ingredients in the smoothie add more green tea if more liquid is needed and blend until smooth. This formula will give energy help reclaim cognitive and memory functions and still provide stable nutrient-rich food imparting a sense of satiety.

Store in a large container in the fridge and make sure to finish all of it over the same day because it will lose some of its healing potency if not consumed on the same day.

Additional Notes

Anxiety radically impairs brain function and clear thinking. So, if you feel anxious during the day, relax and have a Basil Tea (Tulsi Tea) or a green tea with berries for extra flavor. Manuka honey, stevia, and xylitol, or even agave syrup can be used sparingly to sweeten if needed. Remember sugar is a drug that contributes directly to chronic inflammation and can contribute to chronic illnesses, and brain dysfunction, especially excessive intake over long periods.

DAILY SMOOTHIE 02 –"ENERGY BY DAY, GOOD SLEEP BY NIGHT"

(Active & Restful)

This smoothie promotes sustained energy throughout the day. The idea here is that if you have stable balanced energy throughout your day, and you remain active throughout the day, then you avoid long naps during waking hours – which helps prevent disruptions to your sleep at night. This is an amazing smoothie for endurance, especially mental and physical endurance - Think, "sustain".

Ingredients

1½ Bananas

½ cup of lettuce and watercress mixed

½ cup Blueberries (or either of raspberries, strawberries, or black currants)

1 Handful of fresh unsweetened cranberries

¼ cup walnuts

1 tsp maca powder

1 tablespoon Moringa powder (as tea, or leaf extract)

1 tablespoon coconut oil

½ tsp cinnamon powder

1 tsp freshly grated turmeric (ground and dried turmeric powder is ok too)

1 cup green tea (pre-made)

1 cup coconut milk

1 teaspoon flaxseed oil

*½ teaspoon ground black pepper

*(for bio-availability of curcumin in turmeric – leave out if not palatable for you)

Method

First, make a cup of green tea and let it steep while preparing the other ingredients

Wash & soak fruit & greens well for 5 minutes – afterward place straight into a glass blender

Grate the turmeric and add to blender with the balance of the ingredients

Add the green tea to the blender

Blend until smooth and refrigerate for 1 day only

Enjoy your smoothie in between your three main (moderate) meals of your day

Additional Notes

Don't forget you can add any green leafy vegetables such as spinach, lettuce, beet greens, Gotu kola (pennywort) and watercress, sprouts. Also, consider adding 1 tablespoon of chia seeds and/or 1 teaspoon black cumin seed oil to make it extra potent and beneficial for your health.

Final Thoughts

Many of the issues we have discussed in this book have some genealogical elements to them such as genetic predispositions. We get caught up in realizing that our parents and siblings' health may show our own susceptibility to developing neurological and chronic health issues, and often skip the opportunity to look at the whole picture. However, a lot of our neurological health can be managed quite easily whilst preventing any further health issues too all by simply making sure to practice self-discipline, healthy eating habits, and appropriate self-care day by day.

All too often people are told these days that medication is the ONLY path to wellness; though such advice or assertions might be given with the best of intentions it usually leads to the prescription of chemical solutions that *temporarily alleviate symptoms,* often at some cost to unrelated systems in the body via horrific side effects.

Chronic illnesses do NOT respond well to medication in the long term, if they did we wouldn't be seeing the statistics for heart disease, depression, diabetes, cancer, and other chronic diseases of modern living that we do see today. Many symptoms have been alleviated, but not much actual curing or reversal is going on, not in the pharmaceutical chemical prescription sense of health anyway – these medications very often throw us more off-balance in the long run than the symptoms we might have had to deal with without them.

Conventional medical approaches have worked well for some people, in specific and narrow domains, for very specific outcomes and purposes, but it cannot proudly claim to be a successful approach overall when it comes to the inevitably poor health outcomes for chronic degenerative lifestyle disorders – for effective treatments in that sphere, something different is required.

So, even the limited, transient, and narrow applications of medication only really justify such methods as a last resort in specific appropriate circumstances, other forms of care usually do exist and have proven scientific evidence to show they're safer, cheaper, and way more effective – bear this in mind at all times when confronted with opinions to the contrary, the science and epidemiology don't lie – my personal clinical experience stands testimony to the truth of the insufficiency of such approaches when compared to approaches that actually do end up with multiple beneficial outcomes in chronic cases of illness.

By reading this book and applying some of the evidence-based advice, tools, and strategies presented here, you may find your solution is really as simple as changing your diet and supplementing smartly, reducing stress, sleeping properly, and remaining committed, positive, and motivated to take responsibility for your health in a powerful way – prescribed medications are definitely not as effective, reclaim your brain, reclaim your life.

Final Tips:

Set yourself up for success. Having identified the areas where you need to improve then the next step is to do something concrete and practical about those areas! Creating new habits takes a lot of effort and dedication. Take some guesswork out of the process and make it impossible to deviate from that plan. Set up your breakfast options the evening before and lay your clothes out the day before. If you take medication or supplements, consider investing in a pill container that budgets those items throughout the day. It's simple: you will not get very far if things become too tough for you. Don't let that happen.

Don't overwhelm yourself. While it is great to create new habits, these changes take time. It takes at least a month to create a new routine. Do not try to introduce too many changes at once; this will result in burnout and very well may leave you in a worse place than where you began. Similarly, accept that your road will be paved by your mistakes. With that in mind, proceed.

Seek medical help. I spend a good part of this book stressing that medication is not the only journey. However, before changing things up, run them by your doctor first. Make sure you can create these changes in a straightforward, healthy fashion.

Figure out your "why." Why do you care about making this change now? Why is your journey worth finishing? Your answer may include a weight goal or your progress may be dedicated to a spouse, family member, or loved one. Whoever or whatever comes to mind, think of this person every time you create change. You will be propelled forward by your love and desire.

Know your worth. Whatever changes you make, keep your health and well-being in mind.

Methods included in this book are dedicated to clearing neurological illnesses such as memory problems, depression, anxiety, brain fog, and migraines. While family history and other things beyond your control may make you more susceptible to developing these issues, you are responsible for your own fate.

Do not take any of these neurological issues lightly, for they can be signs that more diseases, some of which are incurable, can come out of this. Through regularly choosing foods in the western diet, such as high fructose items, synthetic sweeteners, and gluten, we can destroy our livers and eventually devastate our body's systems. When our stomachs are unhappy, our brains are equally as unhappy. Over time, we risk developing illnesses such as cardiac arrest, stroke, and high blood pressure. These adverse health effects damage the quality of blood that filters to the brain. Additionally, choosing nutrient-barren foods does nothing to help our system of neurotransmitters or the body's messaging system.

While it may be easy to change our diets, it can be harder to change our environment. We may be able to locate fresh fruits, vegetables, and grains, but we may be contractually bound to stay where we are or unable to afford any other home in the area. Leave if you can afford it; if you cannot move, try minimizing your time spent in these areas. Try doing your business in a different area or taking a trip elsewhere instead of spending your time surrounded by toxins.

There are several ways that you can improve yourself and make yourself healthy again while protecting your brain. The onset of cognitive illnesses is quite a terrifying premise for anyone. So, it makes sense to try and avoid them as much as possible. This is possible if you push yourself to become healthier and adopt healthier habits.

Remember, eat healthily, exercise, and remove yourself from potential environmental toxins around you. Those three changes that you can make will ultimately change your lifestyle and make it healthier and you will start protecting your brain in the process.

When I first met our friend Leanne, I instantly knew that she was going to be a difficult case, but I knew that she was already on the road to recovery because she chose to seek help. That is most of the battle won... when you decide to seek help when you know that you need it.

This is just the beginning of your journey, but the fact that you have chosen to read this book is proof that you are already on the road to healing your body and your brain. You should be very proud of yourself for your accomplishments thus far. Just remember to keep your head down and keep going. Once you form these new habits, you will discover how pleasant it is to live a healthier lifestyle.

Your body and your brain are going to thank you for this decision; you have made the choice already, now it is just a simple matter of following through, and then thanking yourself generously.

All the best with your health!

LEAVE A 1-CLICK REVIEW!

Overall rating

Add a photo or video

Shoppers find images and videos more helpful than text alone.

Add a headline

What's most important to know?

Write your review

What did you like or dislike? What did you use this product for?

I would be incredibly thankful if you could just take 60 seconds to write a brief review on Amazon, even if it's just a few sentences.

Click Here to leave a quick review

REFERENCES

1. YOUR BRAIN, YOU, AND YOUR QUALITY OF LIFE

1. World Health Organization. *Neurological disorders: public health challenges*. World Health Organization, 2006. Available at https://www.who.int/mental_health/neurology/neurological_disorders_report_web.pdf?ua
2. Anxiety and Depression Association of America. (n.d.) Facts & Statistics. adaa.org, https://adaa.org/about-adaa/press-room/facts-statistics

2. A CLOSER LOOK AT NEUROTRANSMITTERS

1. Anxiety and Depression Association of America. (n.d.) Facts & Statistics. adaa.org, https://adaa.org/about-adaa/press-room/facts-statistics
2. Anxiety and Depression Association of America. (n.d.) Facts & Statistics. adaa.org, https://adaa.org/about-adaa/press-room/facts-statistics
3. Anxiety and Depression Association of America. (n.d.) Facts & Statistics. adaa.org, https://adaa.org/about-adaa/press-room/facts-statistics
4. Anxiety and Depression Association of America. (n.d.) Facts & Statistics. adaa.org, https://adaa.org/about-adaa/press-room/facts-statistics

3. WHEN THINGS GO WRONG (A)

1. Cutrer F., et al. Pathophysiology, clinical manifestations, and diagnosis of migraine in adults. In: UpToDate, Jerry W Swanson, John F Dashe (Eds), UpToDate, Waltham, MA, 2012.

2. Rizzoli PB. Talking about migraine. Harvard Health Letter. www.health.hardvard.edu. January 2012

3. Charles A. Advances in the basic and clinical science of migraine. Ann Neurol. 2009;65(5):491-498

4. Anxiety and Depression Association of America. (n.d.) Facts & Statistics. adaa.org, https://adaa.org/about-adaa/press-room/facts-statistics

5. Ibid.

6. Nepon, J. (2011). *The Relationship Between Anxiety Disorders and Suicide Attempts: Findings from the National Epidemiological Survey on Alcohol-Related Conditions.* HHS Public Access. 27(9): 791-798. www.ncbi.nlm.nih.gov.

7. Ibid.

8. Ibid.

9. Upadhyaya P, Seth V, Ahmad M. "Therapy for AD: An update." African Journal of Pharmacy and Pharmacology. 4.6 (2010): 408-21.

10. Knopman DS. AD and Other Dementias. In: Goldman L, Schafer AI. Goldman's Cecil Medicine. 24th ed. Philadelphia, PA:Elsevier;2012.

11. Knopman DS. AD and Other Dementias. In: Goldman L, Schafer AI. Goldman's Cecil Medicine. 24th ed. Philadelphia, PA:Elsevier;2012.

12. Tarawneh R, Holtzman DM. "The clinical problem of symptomatic Alzheimer disease and mild cognitive impairment." Cold Spring Harb Perspect Med. 2.5 (2012):a006148.

13. Billingsley, K.J. (2018, March 13). *Genetic Risk Factors in Parkinson's Disease.* National Library of Medicine. 373(1): 9-20. www.pubmed.gov.

14. Sian, J. (n.d). *MPTP-Induced Parkinsonian Syndrome.* Basic Neurochemistry: Molecular, Cellular, and Medical Aspects. 6th edition. https://www.ncbi.nlm.nih.gov/books/NBK27974/

15. National Institute on Aging. (n.d.). What is Alzheimer's Disease? nia.nih.gov, https://www.nia.nih.gov/health/what-alzheimers-disease.

16. Anxiety and Depression Association of America. (n.d.) Facts & Statistics. adaa.org, https://adaa.org/about-adaa/press-room/facts-statistics

17. Kanoski, J. Scott, E. Davidson, F. Terry, L. (2012, April 18). Western Diet Consumption and Cognitive Impairment: Links to Hippocampal Dysfunction and Obesity. Health and Human Services Public Access. https://www.ncbi.nlm.nih.gov/pmc/articles/PMC3056912/

18. Wint, C. (2018). *Diabetic Neuropathy: Treatment, Symptoms, and Causes.* www.healthline.com

19. Wint, C. (2018). *Diabetic Neuropathy: Treatment, Symptoms, and Causes.* www.healthline.com

20. Leech, J. (2017). *10 Delicious Herbs and Spices with Powerful Health Benefits.* Evidence Based Nutrition. www.healthline.com.

21. Billingsley, K.J. (2018, March 13). *Genetic Risk Factors in Parkinson's Disease.* National Library of Medicine. 373(1): 9-20. www.pubmed.gov.

22. Sian, J. (n.d). *MPTP-Induced Parkinsonian Syndrome.* Basic Neurochemistry: Molecular, Cellular, and Medical Aspects. 6th edition. https://www.ncbi.nlm.nih.gov/books/NBK27974/

23. Billingsley, K.J. (2018, March 13). *Genetic Risk Factors in Parkinson's Disease.* National Library of Medicine. 373(1): 9-20. www.pubmed.gov.

24. Billingsley, K.J. (2018, March 13). *Genetic Risk Factors in Parkinson's Disease.* National Library of Medicine. 373(1): 9-20. www.pubmed.gov.

25. Sian, J. (n.d). *MPTP-Induced Parkinsonian Syndrome.* Basic Neurochemistry: Molecular, Cellular, and Medical Aspects. 6th edition. https://www.ncbi.nlm.nih.gov/books/NBK27974/

4. WHEN THINGS GO WRONG (B)

1. World Health Organization. *Neurological disorders: public health challenges.* World Health Organization, 2006. Available at https://www.who.int/mental_health/neurology/neurological_disorders_report_web.pdf?ua

2. Anxiety and Depression Association of America. (n.d.) Facts & Statistics. adaa.org, https://adaa.org/about-adaa/press-room/facts-statistics

3. Rizzoli PB. Talking about migraine. Harvard Health Letter. www.health.hardvard.edu. January 2012

4. Charles A. Advances in the basic and clinical science of migraine. Ann Neurol. 2009;65(5):491-498

5. Cutrer F., et al. Pathophysiology, clinical manifestations, and diagnosis of migraine in adults. In: UpToDate, Jerry W Swanson, John F Dashe (Eds), UpToDate, Waltham, MA, 2012.

6. Gallagher, M., (2012) Chapter 1: Symptomatic Care Pending Diagnosis (pg. 1). In: Bope, E. (Ed.), Conn's Current Therapy 2012 (1st ed.). Saunders, An Imprint of Elsevier.

7. Fukui PT, GonçalvesTR, Strabelli CG, et al. Trigger factors in migraine patients. Arq Neuropsiquiatr. 2008;66(3A):494-9.

8. Braun, E., (2010) Chapter 17: Pain Management in the Head and Neck Patient (pg. 246). In: Flint, P. (Ed.), Cummings Otolaryngology: Head & Neck Surgery (5th ed.). Mosby, An Imprint of Elsevier

9. Gallagher, M., (2012) Chapter 1: Symptomatic Care Pending Diagnosis (pg. 1). In: Bope, E. (Ed.), Conn's Current Therapy 2012 (1st ed.). Saunders, An Imprint of Elsevier.

10. Fukui PT, GonçalvesTR, Strabelli CG, et al. Trigger factors in migraine patients. Arq Neuropsiquiatr. 2008;66(3A):494-9.

11. Lipton RB, Gobel H, Einhaupl KM, Wilks K, Mauskop A. Petasiteshybridus root (butterbur) is an effective preventive treatment for migraine. Neurology. 2004;63(12):2240-2244

12. Ibid.

13. Ibid.

14. Mijalski C, Dakay K, Miller-Patterson C, Saad A, Silver B, Khan M. Magnesium for Treatment of Reversible Cerebral Vasoconstriction Syndrome: Case Series. *The Neurohospitalist.* Jul 2016;6(3):111-113

15. Li W, Zheng T, Altura BM, Altura BT. Sex steroid hormones exert biphasic effects on cytosolic magnesium ions in cerebral vascu- lar smooth muscle cells: possible relationships to migraine frequency in premenstrual syndromes and stroke incidence. Brain Res Bull. 2001 Jan 1;54(1)

16. Ross SM. Clinical applications of integrative therapies for prevention and treatment of migraine headaches. Holist NursPract. 2011;25(1):49-52

17. Ross SM. Coenzyme q10: ubiquinone: a potent antioxidant and key energy facilitator for the heart. Holist NursPract. 2007;21(4):213-214

5. EXPOSURE!

1. Cannon, Jason R., and J. Timothy Greenamyre. "The role of environmental exposures in neurodegeneration and neurodegenerative diseases." *Toxicological Sciences* 124.2 (2011): 225-250.

6. HAPPY GUT, HAPPY BRAIN, HAPPY YOU!

1. Sender, Ron, et al. "Revised Estimates for the Number of Human and Bacteria Cells in the Body." New Results (2016): 36103.

2. Bianconi, Eva, et al. "An estimation of the number of cells in the human body." Annals of Human Biology 40.6 (2013): 463–471.

3. Saey, Tina Hesman. "Body's Bacteria Don't Outnumber Human Cells so Much After All." Microbiology, Physiology. Science News, Mar. 2016.

4. Saey, Tina Hesman. "The Vast Virome."Microbes,Ecosystems,Health. Science News, 18 Nov. 2016.

5. Milliken, Grennan. ARE VIRUSES ALIVE? NEW EVIDENCE SAYS YES. Popular Science (Web Based) 2016.

6. Neu, Josef, and Jona Rushing. "Cesarean Versus Vaginal Delivery: Long Term Infant Outcomes and the Hygiene Hypothesis." 38.2 : Web Based. 28 Nov. 2016.

7. Ibid.

8. "Exploring the role of gut bacteria in digestion."(2010)

9. Ramakrishna, BS. "Role of the Gut Microbiota in Human Nutrition and Metabolism."Journal of gastroenterology and hepatology. 28. (2013): 9–17.

10. Ibid.

11. Bäckhed, F, et al. "The Gut Microbiota as an Environmental Factor That Regulates Fat Storage." Proceedings of the National Academy of Sciences of the United States of America. 101.44 (2004): 15718–23.

12. Carabotti, Marilia, et al. "The Gut-Brain Axis: Interactions Between Enteric Microbiota, Central and Enteric Nervous Systems."Central and Enteric Nervous Systems." (2015)

13. Ibid.

14. Ramakrishna, BS. "Role of the Gut Microbiota in Human Nutrition and Metabolism."Journal of gastroenterology and hepatology. 28. (2013): 9–17.

15. Ibid.

16. Belkaid, Yasmine, and Timothy Hand."Role of the Microbiota in Immunity and Inflammation." 157.1 (2014):

17. Kau, Andrew, et al. "Human Nutrition, the Gut Microbiome, and Immune System: Envisioning the Future." Nature (2011): 327–226.

18. Neu, Josef, and Jona Rushing. "Cesarean Versus Vaginal Delivery: Long Term Infant Outcomes and the Hygiene Hypothesis." 38.2 (Web based)

19. Mueller, Noel T., et al. "The Infant Microbiome Development: Mom Matters." 21.2 (2014)

20. "Your Changing Microbiome." Web Based. 19Nov. 2016.

21. Dominguez-Bello, MG, et al. "Delivery Mode Shapes the Acquisition and Structure of the Initial Microbiota Across Multiple Body Habi-

tats in Newborns." Proceedings of the National Academy of Sciences of the United States of America. 107.26 (2010): 11971–5.

22. Ibid.

23. MacIntyre, David A., et al. "The Vaginal Microbiome During Pregnancy and the Postpartum Period in a European Population." (2015)

24. Ibid.

25. Filippo, De, et al. "Impact of Diet in Shaping Gut Microbiota Revealed by a Comparative Study in Children from Europe and Rural Africa." Proceedings of the National Academy of Sciences of the United States of America. 107.33 (2010): 14691–6.

26. Conlon, Michael A., and Anthony R. Bird."The Impact of Diet and Lifestyle on Gut Microbiota and Human Health." 7.1 (2014)

27. Eske, J. (2019). *Leaky Gut Syndrome: What It Is, Symptoms, and Treatments.* Newsletter. www.medicalnewstoday.com.

28. Eske, J. (2019). *Leaky Gut Syndrome: What It Is, Symptoms, and Treatments.* Newsletter. www.medicalnewstoday.com.

29. Kanoski, J. Scott, E. Davidson, F. Terry, L. (2012, April 18). Western Diet Consumption and Cognitive Impairment: Links to Hippocampal Dysfunction and Obesity. Health and Human Services Public Access. https://www.ncbi.nlm.nih.gov/pmc/articles/PMC3056912/

30. Anxiety and Depression Association of America. (n.d.) Facts & Statistics. adaa.org, https://adaa.org/about-adaa/press-room/facts-statistics

31. Eske, J. (2019). *Leaky Gut Syndrome: What It Is, Symptoms, and Treatments.* Newsletter. www.medicalnewstoday.com.

32. Eske, J. (2019). *Leaky Gut Syndrome: What It Is, Symptoms, and Treatments.* Newsletter. www.medicalnewstoday.com.

33. Leech, J. (2017). *10 Delicious Herbs and Spices with Powerful Health Benefits.* Evidence Based Nutrition. www.healthline.com.

34. Kanoski, J. Scott, E. Davidson, F. Terry, L. (2012, April 18). Western Diet Consumption and Cognitive Impairment: Links to Hippocampal Dysfunction and Obesity. Health and Human Services Public Access. https://www.ncbi.nlm.nih.gov/pmc/articles/PMC3056912/

7. SLEEP, EXERCISE, STRESS & ANXIETY

1. http://link.springer.com/article/10.1007/BF02146962
2. http://link.springer.com/chapter/10.1007/978-1-4613-4609-8_8
3. http://www.jbc.org/content/242/9/2278.short
4. http://www.biochemsoctrans.org/content/35/5/1295
5. Ibid.
6. http://www.nejm.org/doi/full/10.1056/nejm200002173420702
7. http://www.sciencedirect.com/science/article/pii/S0001691802001348
8. http://onlinelibrary.wiley.com/doi/10.1111/j.1460-9568.2008.06524.x/full
9. http://bjsm.bmj.com/content/43/1/25.short
10. http://www.sciencedirect.com/science/article/pii/S1552526009000600
11. https://www.ncbi.nlm.nih.gov/pmc/articles/PMC4111643/
12. http://circ.ahajournals.org/content/107/1/e2
13. http://ijmpo.org/article.asp?issn=0971-5851;year=2009;volume=30;issue=2;spage=61;epage=70;aulast=Rajarajeswaran
14. http://care.diabetesjournals.org/content/27/suppl_1/s58.full
15. .https://www.researchgate.net/profile/Pierpaolo_De_Feo/publication/6865754_Exercise_and_diabetes/links/0c960525a4df315c59000000.pdf
16. .https://www.researchgate.net/profile/Stuart_Chipkin/publication/222895939_Exercise_and_diabetes/links/544565b90cf22b3c14dde5a3.pdf
17. http://onlinelibrary.wiley.com/doi/10.1002/j.1550-8528.1993.tb00603.x/abstract
18. http://onlinelibrary.wiley.com/doi/10.1002/ana.22096/full
19. http://www.sciencedirect.com/science/article/pii/S0149763405001508
20. https://www.ncbi.nlm.nih.gov/pmc/articles/PMC4111643/

21. http://www.udptclinic.comjournalclub/noajc/11-12/November/04%20Ebersbach%20LSVT%20BIG,%202010%20(1).pdf

22. http://www.sciencedirect.com/science/article/pii/S1389945710002868

23. http://onlinelibrary.wiley.com/doi/10.1111/j.1479-8425.2006.00235.x/full

24. http://www.scielo.br/scielo.php?pid=S1807-59322012000600017&script=sci_arttext

25. http://www.greenmedinfo.com/article/combination-exercise-training-resulted-improvements-cardiovascular-risk-profil

26. http://circ.ahajournals.org/content/116/5/572.short

27. Tawakol, Ahmed, et al. "Relation between resting amygdalar activity and cardiovascular events: a longitudinal and cohort study." *The Lancet* 389.10071 (2017): 834-845.

28. https://www.sciencedaily.com/releases/2017/01/170111213656.htm

29. Ibid.

30. http://articles.mercola.com/sites/articles/archive/2015/12/17/stress-makes-you-sick.aspx

31. http://www.thedoctorwillseeyounow.com/content/stress/art2861.html

32. http://articles.mercola.com/sites/articles/archive/2015/12/17/stress-makes-you-sick.aspx

33. http://operationmeditation.com/discover/increase-serotonin-naturally-in-5-easy-ways/

34. https://draxe.com/cortisol-levels/

35. https://www.ncbi.nlm.nih.gov/pubmed/26254769

36. https://www.ncbi.nlm.nih.gov/pubmed/27103058

37. https://www.ncbi.nlm.nih.gov/pubmed/27840104

38. https://www.ncbi.nlm.nih.gov/pubmed/20855902

39. http://www.businessinsider.com/power-poses-interview-body-language-2014-3

40. Zhang J, Ma RC et al. Relationship of Sleep Quantity and Quality with 24-Hour Urinary Catecholamines and Salivary Awakening Cortisol in Healthy Middle-Aged Adults. Sleep, 2011; 34(2): 225-233.

41. Bonnet MH and Arand DL. Hyperarousal and Insomnia: State of the Science. Sleep Medicine Reviews, 2010;14:9-15

42. Butcher SK, Killampalli V, Lascelles D, et al. Raised cortisol:DHEAS ratios in the elderly after injury: potential impact upon neutrophil function and immunity. Aging Cell. 2005 4(6):319-24.

43. Chiodini I, Scillitani A. Role of cortisol hypersecretion in the pathogenesis of osteoporosis. RecentiProg Med. 2008 99(6):309-13.

44. Duong M, Cohen JI, and Convit A. h cortisol levels are associated with low quality food choice in type 2 diabetes. Endocrine. 2012 41(1):76-81.

45. Irwin MR, Wang M et al. Sleep Deprivation and Activation of Morning Levels of Cellular and Genomic Markers of Inflammation. Archives of Internal Medicine, 2006; 166: 1756-1762.

46. Smith MT, Quartana PJ et al. Mechanisms By Which Sleep Disturbance Contributes to Osteoarthritic Pain: A Conceptual Model. Current Pain and Headache Reports, 2009; 13: 447-54.

47. UAB News. [Lollar J.] Sleep debt hikes risk of stroke symptoms despite healthy BMI. 6/11/2012 Available at: http://www.uab.edu/news/latest/item/2483-sleep-debt-hikes-risk-of-stroke-symptoms-despite-healthy-bmi?tmpl=component&print=1   Accessed 03/01/2017

48. Chien KL, Chen PC, Hsu HC, et al. Habitual sleep duration and insomnia and the risk of cardiovascular events and all-cause death: report from a community-based cohort. Sleep. 2010 33(2):177-84.

49. Hublin C, Partinen M, Koskenvuo M, et al. Heritability and mortality risk of insomnia-related symptoms: a genetic epidemiologic study in a population-based twin cohort. Sleep. 2011 34(7):957-64.

50. http://news.harvard.edu/gazette/story/2011/01/eight-weeks-to-a-better-brain

51. http://www.ahc.umn.edu/img/assets/20825/MindfulnessADHD-Zylowska_et_al.pdf

52. Z Bai, J Chang, C Chen, P Li, K Yang and I Chi. (2015). "Investigating the effect of transcendental meditation on blood pressure: a systematic review and meta-analysis", Journal of Human Hypertension.

53. Brook, Robert D. et al., "Beyond Medications and Diet: Alternative Approaches to Lowering Blood Pressure. A Scientific Statement from the American Heart Association", published on April 22, 2013

54. http://tmhome.com/wp-content/uploads/2012/07/Study-on-stress-reduction-and-mortality.pdf

55. Duraimani S, Schneider RH, Randall OS, Nidich SI, Xu S, Ketete M, et al. (2015) "Effects of Lifestyle Modification on Telomerase Gene Expression in Hypertensive Patients: A Pilot Trial of Stress Reduction and Health Education Programs in African Americans." PLOS ONE 10(11): e0142689. doi:10.1371/journal.pone.0142689

56. https://www.google.com/amp/www.goodtherapy.org/blog/can-listening-to-binaural-beats-make-you-feel-better-0724124/amp/

57. http://gretchenrubin.com/happiness_project/2011/01/six-questions-to-help-you-keep-your-cool-instead-of-losing-your-temper/

58. Anxiety and Depression Association of America. (n.d.) Facts & Statistics. adaa.org, https://adaa.org/about-adaa/press-room/facts-statistics

59. Anxiety and Depression Association of America. (n.d.) Facts & Statistics. adaa.org, https://adaa.org/about-adaa/press-room/facts-statistics

8. NATURAL SUPPLEMENTS & SUPER-FOODS TO HEAL, PROTECT, AND BOOST YOUR BRAIN

1. Xu, Bei, et al. "Luteolin promotes long-term potentiation and improves cognitive functions in chronic cerebral hypoperfused rats." *European journal of pharmacology* 627.1 (2010): 99-105.

2. Liu, Rui, et al. "Luteolin isolated from the medicinal plant Elsholtzia rugulosa (Labiatae) prevents copper-mediated toxicity in β-amyloid precursor protein Swedish mutation overexpressing SH-SY5Y cells." *Molecules* 16.3 (2011): 2084-2096.

3. http://www.mdpi.com/1422-0067/15/1/895/htm

4. http://www.ingentaconnect.com/content/ben/cmc/2011/00000018/00000026/art00011

5. Beal, M. Flint. "Mitochondrial dysfunction and oxidative damage in Alzheimer's and Parkinson's diseases and coenzyme Q10 as a potential treatment." *Journal of bioenergetics and biomembranes* 36.4 (2004): 381-386.

6. Yang, Xifei, et al. "Coenzyme Q10 attenuates β-amyloid pathology in the aged transgenic mice with Alzheimer presenilin 1 mutation." *Journal of Molecular Neuroscience* 34.2 (2008): 165-171.

7. http://content.iospress.com/articles/journal-of-alzheimers-disease/jad110209

8. http://www.ingentaconnect.com/content/ben/cdt/2010/00000011/00000001/art00014

9. Clarke, Robert, et al. "Folate, vitamin B12, and serum total homocysteine levels in confirmed Alzheimer disease." *Archives of neurology* 55.11 (1998): 1449-1455.

10. http://www.pnas.org/content/110/23/9523.short

11. http://journals.plos.org/plosone/article?id=10.1371/journal.pone.0012244

12. Tucker, Katherine L., et al. "High homocysteine and low B vitamins predict cognitive decline in aging men: the Veterans Affairs Normative Aging Study." *The American journal of clinical nutrition* 82.3 (2005): 627-635.

13. http://www.nejm.org/doi/full/10.1056/nejmoa060900

14. http://www.sciencedirect.com/science/article/pii/S0091743504002361

15. http://www.nejm.org/doi/full/10.1056/NEJM198806303182604

16. Institute of Medicine. Food and Nutrition Board. Dietary Reference Intakes: Thiamin, Riboflavin, Niacin, Vitamin B6, Folate, Vitamin B12, Pantothenic Acid, Biotin, and Choline. Washington, DC: National Academy Press, 1998.

17. https://ods.od.nih.gov/factsheets/VitaminB12-HealthProfessional/

18. Riggs, Karen M., et al. "Relations of vitamin B-12, vitamin B-6, folate, and homocysteine to cognitive performance in the Normative

Aging Study." *The American journal of clinical nutrition* 63.3 (1996): 306-314.

19. http://onlinelibrary.wiley.com/doi/10.1111/j.1432-1033.1994.tb18577.x/full

20. http://www.lifestreamrx.com/assets/DouglasDataSheets/PYP.pdf

21. http://www.neurology.org/content/56/9/1188.1.short

22. Kruman, Inna I., et al. "Folic acid deficiency and homocysteine impair DNA repair in hippocampal neurons and sensitize them to amyloid toxicity in experimental models of Alzheimer's disease." *Journal of Neuroscience* 22.5 (2002): 1752-1762.

23. Das, Undurti N. "Folic acid and polyunsaturated fatty acids improve cognitive function and prevent depression, dementia, and Alzheimer's disease—But how and why?." *Prostaglandins, Leukotrienes and Essential Fatty Acids* 78.1 (2008): 11-19.

24. https://ods.od.nih.gov/factsheets/Folate-Consumer/

25. Morris, Martha C., et al. "Dietary niacin and the risk of incident Alzheimer's disease and of cognitive decline." *Journal of Neurology, Neurosurgery & Psychiatry* 75.8 (2004): 1093-1099.

26. http://www.nejm.org/doi/full/10.1056/nejmoa011090

27. Contiguglia, SebastianR, et al. "Total-body magnesium excess in chronic renal failure." *The Lancet* 299.7764 (1972): 1300-1302.

28. Reinhart, Richard A. "Magnesium metabolism: a review with special reference to the relationship between intracellular content and serum levels." *Archives of internal medicine* 148.11 (1988): 2415-2420.

29. Laires, Maria José, Cristina Paula Monteiro, and Manuel Bicho. "Role of cellular magnesium in health and human disease." *Front Biosci* 9.262 (2004): 76.

30. http://onlinelibrary.wiley.com/doi/10.1111/j.1532-5415.1987.tb04664.x/full

31. Kiss, B., and E. Karpati. "Mechanism of action of vinpocetine." *Acta pharmaceutica Hungarica* 66.5 (1996): 213-224.

32. Hagiwara, Masatoshi, Toyoshi Endo, and Hiroyoshi Hidaka. "Effects of vinpocetine on cyclic nucleotide metabolism in vascular smooth muscle." *Biochemical pharmacology* 33.3 (1984): 453-457.

33. http://www.sciencedirect.com/science/article/pii/S092982660200006X

34. DeNoble, Victor J., et al. "Vinpocetine: nootropic effects on scopolamine-induced and hypoxia-induced retrieval deficits of a step-through passive avoidance response in rats." *Pharmacology Biochemistry and Behavior* 24.4 (1986): 1123-1128.

35. http://journals.lww.com/intclinpsychopharm/abstract/1991/00610/efficacy_and_tolerance_of_vinpocetine_in_ambulant.5.aspx

36. Erdman, John, Maria Oria, and Laura Pillsbury. "Eicosapentaenoic Acid (EPA) and Docosahexaenoic Acid (DHA)." (2011).

37. .http://nonamenutrition.com/ns/DisplayMonograph.asp?StoreID=EXMVRHM35QFW8N06361K08Q58P2679H3&DocID=bottomline-docosahexaenoicacid

38. Guesnet, Philippe, and Jean-Marc Alessandri. "Docosahexaenoic acid (DHA) and the developing central nervous system (CNS)–Implications for dietary recommendations." *Biochimie* 93.1 (2011): 7-12.

39. http://link.springer.com/article/10.1007/s00114-003-0470-z

40. Engler, M. M., et al. "Docosahexaenoic acid restores endothelial function in children with hyperlipidemia: results from the EARLY study." *International journal of clinical pharmacology and therapeutics* 42.12 (2004): 672-679.

41. Horrocks, Lloyd A., and Young K. Yeo. "Health benefits of docosahexaenoic acid (DHA)." *Pharmacological Research* 40.3 (1999): 211-225.

42. http://journals.lww.com/annalsofsurgery/Abstract/2009/03000/Enteral_Nutrition_Enriched_With_Eicosapentaenoic.1.aspx

43. http://umm.edu/health/medical/altmed/supplement/alphalipoic-acid

44. http://www.greenmedinfo.com/article/alpha-lipoic-acid-could-be-therapeutic-agent-because-its-inhibitory-effects

45. Hagen, Tory M., et al. "(R)-α-Lipoic acid-supplemented old rats have improved mitochondrial function, decreased oxidative damage, and increased metabolic rate." *The FASEB Journal* 13.2 (1999): 411-418.

46. Long, Jiangang, et al. "Mitochondrial decay in the brains of old rats: ameliorating effect of alpha-lipoic acid and acetyl-L-carnitine." *Neurochemical research* 34.4 (2009): 755-763.

47. http://s3.amazonaws.com/academia.edu.documents/44487871/Alpha_lipoic_acid_a_new_treatment_for_ne20160406-21123-1jb59nd.pdf?AWSAccessKeyId=AKIAJ56TQJRTWSMTNPEA&Expires=1481197913&Signature=VruwDM6By42WaA1svjdqoNjEtcY%3D&response-content-disposition=inline%3B%20filename%3DAlpha_lipoic_acid_a_new_treatment_for_ne.pdf#page=16

48. Liu, F., et al. "Curative effect of alpha-lipoic acid on peripheral neuropathy in type 2 diabetes: a clinical study." *Zhonghua yi xue za zhi* 87.38 (2007): 2706-2709.

49. http://www.greenmedinfo.com/article/alpha-lipoic-acid-and-gamma-linolenic-acid-significantly-improve-symptom-scores-and

50. https://scholar.google.co.za/scholar?q=Lipoic+acid+down-regulates+inflammation+in+multiple+sclerosis+patients.&btnG=&hl=en&as_sdt=1%2C5

51. http://www.greenmedinfo.com/article/alpha-lipoic-appears-be-effective-neuroprotective-agent-alzheimers-disease

52. Melli, Giorgia, et al. "Alpha-lipoic acid prevents mitochondrial damage and neurotoxicity in experimental chemotherapy neuropathy." *Experimental neurology* 214.2 (2008): 276-284.

53. http://www.greenmedinfo.com/article/alpha-lipoic-acid-prevents-mitochondrial-damage-and-neurotoxicity-experimental

54. http://www.greenmedinfo.com/article/alpha-lipoic-may-have-profound-therapeutic-role-treatment-pancreatic-cancer

55. Li, Donghui. "Diabetes and pancreatic cancer." *Molecular carcinogenesis* 51.1 (2012): 64-74.

56. Salinthone, Sonemany, et al. "Lipoic acid stimulates cAMP production via G protein-coupled receptor-dependent and-independent mechanisms." *The Journal of nutritional biochemistry* 22.7 (2011): 681-690.

57. https://www.ncbi.nlm.nih.gov/pmc/articles/PMC3072460/

58. http://www.biomedsearch.com/article/Mercury-toxicity-antioxidants-part-role/96416600.html

59. Gauthier, Eric, et al. "Aluminum forms in drinking water and risk of Alzheimer's disease." *Environmental research* 84.3 (2000): 234-246.

60. http://www.greenmedinfo.com/article/combination-vitamin-e-vitamin-c-alpha-lipoic-acid-and-stilbene-resveratrol

61. http://www.greenmedinfo.com/article/lipoic-acid-mitigates-bisphenol-induced-testicular-mitochondrial-toxicity-rats

62. http://tih.sagepub.com/content/29/10/875.short

63. McMackin, Craig J., et al. "Effect of Combined Treatment With α-Lipoic Acid and Acetyl-L-Carnitine on Vascular Function and Blood Pressure in Patients With Coronary Artery Disease." *The Journal of Clinical Hypertension* 9.4 (2007): 249-255.

64. http://www.fasebj.org/content/15/3/700.short

65. Hagen, Tory M., et al. "Mitochondrial decay in the aging rat heart." *Annals of the New York Academy of Sciences* 959.1 (2002): 491-507.

66. http://www.greenmedinfo.com/article/lipoic-acid-down-regulates-inflammation-multiple-sclerosis-patients

67. Sun-Edelstein, Christina, and Alexander Mauskop. "Alternative headache treatments: nutraceuticals, behavioral and physical treatments." *Headache: The Journal of Head and Face Pain* 51.3 (2011): 469-483.

68. http://onlinelibrary.wiley.com/doi/10.1111/j.1526-4610.2011.01846.x/full

69. http://www.greenmedinfo.com/article/alpha-lipoic-acid-had-ameliorative-effects-against-hfcs-induced-pancreatic

70. Topsakal, Senay, et al. "Alpha lipoic acid attenuates high-fructose-induced pancreatic toxicity." *Pancreatology* 16.3 (2016): 347-352.

71. http://www.nature.com/nature/journal/v278/n5706/abs/278737a0.html

72. Kalt, Wilhelmina, et al. "Antioxidant capacity, vitamin C, phenolics, and anthocyanins after fresh storage of small fruits." *Journal of Agricultural and Food Chemistry* 47.11 (1999): 4638-4644.

73. http://circ.ahajournals.org/content/99/9/1156.short

74. Levine, Mark, et al. "Criteria and recommendations for vitamin C intake." *Jama* 281.15 (1999): 1415-1423.

75. Morris, Martha Clare, et al. "Relation of the tocopherol forms to incident Alzheimer disease and to cognitive change." *The American journal of clinical nutrition* 81.2 (2005): 508-514.

76. http://www.fasebj.org/content/17/8/816.short

77. Kuo, Fonghsu, et al. "Nanoemulsions of an anti-oxidant synergy formulation containing gamma tocopherol have enhanced bioavailability and anti-inflammatory properties." *International journal of pharmaceutics* 363.1 (2008): 206-213.

78. Hensley, Kenneth, et al. "Reactive oxygen species, cell signaling, and cell injury." *Free Radical Biology and Medicine* 28.10 (2000): 1456-1462.

79. http://www.karger.com/Article/Abstract/134382

80. http://content.iospress.com/articles/journal-of-alzheimers-disease/jad101986

81. http://content.iospress.com/articles/journal-of-alzheimers-disease/jad110560

82. https://www.jstage.jst.go.jp/article/tjem/212/3/212_3_275/_article

83. Wilkins, Consuelo H., et al. "Vitamin D deficiency is associated with low mood and worse cognitive performance in older adults." *The American Journal of Geriatric Psychiatry* 14.12 (2006): 1032-1040.

84. http://www.neurology.org/content/83/10/920.short

85. Chapuy, Marie C., et al. "Vitamin D3 and calcium to prevent hip fractures in elderly women." *New England journal of medicine* 327.23 (1992): 1637-1642.

86. http://www.biochemsoctrans.org/content/33/4/573.abstract

87. Wion, D., et al. "1, 25-Dihydroxyvitamin D3 is a potent inducer of nerve growth factor synthesis." *Journal of neuroscience research* 28.1 (1991): 110-114.

88. Kalueff, A. V., K. O. Eremin, and P. Tuohimaa. "Mechanisms of neuroprotective action of vitamin D3." *Biochemistry (Moscow)* 69.7 (2004): 738-741.

89. http://www.webmd.com/vitamins-supplements/ingredientmono-834-acetyl-l-carnitine.aspx?activeingredientid=834&activeingredientname=acetyl-l-carnitine

90. http://www.neurology.org/content/41/11/1726.short

91. http://www.juvenon.com/pdfs/AC_Meta-analysis_paper.pdf

92. http://care.diabetesjournals.org/content/28/1/89.short

93. http://www.greenmedinfo.com/article/acetyl-l-carnitine-exhibits-pain-killing-activity-animal-model-neuropathy

94. http://www.greenmedinfo.com/article/acetyl-l-carnitine-has-therapeutic-effect-symptomatic-treatment-antiretroviral-toxic

95. http://www.greenmedinfo.com/article/acetyl-l-carnitine-has-positive-long-term-effect-treatment-antiretroviral-toxic-neuropathy

96. Bianchi, Giulia, et al. "Symptomatic and neurophysiological responses of paclitaxel-or cisplatin-induced neuropathy to oral acetyl-L-carnitine." *European Journal of Cancer* 41.12 (2005): 1746-1750.

97. http://www.greenmedinfo.com/article/combination-mitochondrial-targeting-nutrients-may-improve-skeletal-mitochondrial-dysfunction

98. https://www.researchgate.net/profile/Jay_Pettegrew/publication/12203290_Acetyl-L-carnitine_physical-chemical_metabolic_and_therapeutic_properties_Relevance_for_its_mode_of_action_in_Alzheimer%27s_disease_and_geriatric_depression/links/568a96bb08aebccc4e1a0a71.pdf

99. Brevetti, Gregorio, et al. "Muscle carnitine deficiency in patients with severe peripheral vascular disease." *Circulation* 84.4 (1991): 1490-1495.

100. .http://s3.amazonaws.com/academia.edu.documents/43660393/agradoc144.pdf?AWSAccessKeyId=AKIAJ56TQJRTWSMTNPEA&Expires=1481186721&Signature=g1ztdPeA552cWyYwG%2BE1e5GiEZQ%3D&response-content-disposition=inline%3B%20filename%3DPlacebo-controlled_double-blind_randomiz.pdf

101. http://www.telegraph.co.uk/news/health/news/6250641/Extra-virgin-olive-oil-could-prevent-Alzheimers-disease.html

102. Martín-Peláez, Sandra, et al. "Health effects of olive oil polyphenols: recent advances and possibilities for the use of health claims." *Molecular nutrition & food research* 57.5 (2013): 760-771.

103. Kostomoiri, Myrta, et al. "Oleuropein, an anti-oxidant polyphenol constituent of olive promotes α-secretase cleavage of the amyloid precursor protein (AβPP)." *Cellular and molecular neurobiology* 33.1 (2013): 147-154.

104. Abuznait, Alaa H., et al. "Olive-oil-derived oleocanthal enhances β-amyloid clearance as a potential neuroprotective mechanism against Alzheimer's disease: in vitro and in vivo studies." *ACS chemical neuroscience* 4.6 (2013): 973-982.

105. http://www.ingentaconnect.com/content/ben/car/2011/00000008/00000005/art00009

106. Pitt, Jason, et al. "Alzheimer's-associated Aβ oligomers show altered structure, immunoreactivity and synaptotoxicity with low doses of oleocanthal." *Toxicology and applied pharmacology* 240.2 (2009): 189-197.

107. http://content.iospress.com/articles/journal-of-alzheimers-disease/jad110662

108. Li, Wenkai, et al. "Inhibition of tau fibrillization by oleocanthal via reaction with the amino groups of tau." *Journal of neurochemistry* 110.4 (2009): 1339-1351.

109. Covas, María-Isabel. "Olive oil and the cardiovascular system." *Pharmacological Research* 55.3 (2007): 175-186.

110. http://nutritionreviews.oxfordjournals.org/content/56/5/142.abstract

111. http://coconutresearchcenter.org/wp-content/uploads/2015/11/Fernando_et-al_2015.pdf

112. Boudrault, Cynthia, Richard P. Bazinet, and David WL Ma. "Experimental models and mechanisms underlying the protective effects of n-3 polyunsaturated fatty acids in Alzheimer's disease." *The Journal of nutritional biochemistry* 20.1 (2009): 1-10.

113. Sadeghi, S., F. A. Wallace, and P. C. Calder. "Dietary lipids modify the cytokine response to bacterial lipopolysaccharide in mice." *IMMUNOLOGY-OXFORD-* 96 (1999): 404-410.

114. Intahphuak, S., P. Khonsung, and A. Panthong. "Anti-inflammatory, analgesic, and antipyretic activities of virgin coconut oil." *Pharmaceutical Biology* 48.2 (2010): 151-157.

115. Sellappan, Subramani, Casimir C. Akoh, and Gerard Krewer. "Phenolic compounds and antioxidant capacity of Georgia-grown blueberries and blackberries." *Journal of Agricultural and Food Chemistry* 50.8 (2002): 2432-2438.

116. http://www.eurohealth-spain.com/articulos/disease.pdf

117. Wang, Shiow Y., and Hsin-Shan Lin. "Antioxidant activity in fruits and leaves of blackberry, raspberry, and strawberry varies with cultivar and developmental stage." *Journal of agricultural and food chemistry* 48.2 (2000): 140-146.

118. http://nutritionreviews.oxfordjournals.org/content/68/3/168.abstract

119. Shukitt-Hale B, Carey AN, Jenkins D, Rabin BM, Joseph JA. Beneficial effects of fruit extracts on neuronal function and behavior in a rodent model of accelerated aging. Neurobiol Aging. 2007 Aug;28(8):1187-94.

120. Kumari, Archana, et al. "Pomegranate (Punica granatum)—Overview." *Int. J. Pharm. Chem. Sci* 1 (2012): 1218-1222.

121. Li, Jun, Fujun Zhang, and Shaohua Wang. "A polysaccharide from pomegranate peels induces the apoptosis of human osteosarcoma cells via the mitochondrial apoptotic pathway." *Tumor Biology* 35.8 (2014): 7475-7482.

122. http://cancerres.aacrjournals.org/content/67/7/3475.short

123. Kim ND, Mehta R, Yu W, et al. Chemopreventive and adjuvant therapeutic potential of pomegranate (Punica Granatum) for human breast cancer. Breast Cancer Res Treat. 2002 Feb;71(3):203-17.

124. Shiraishi, Ryosuke, et al. "Conjugated linoleic acid suppresses colon carcinogenesis in azoxymethane-pretreated rats with long-term feeding of diet containing beef tallow." *Journal of gastroenterology* 45.6 (2010): 625-635.

125. Zou, Xuan, et al. "Mitochondrial dysfunction in obesity-associated nonalcoholic fatty liver disease: the protective effects of pomegranate

with its active component punicalagin." *Antioxidants & redox signaling* 21.11 (2014): 1557-1570.

126. http://www.lifeextension.com/magazine/2010/5/is-conventional-pomegranate-extract-enough/page-02?p=1

127. .https://www.joinultimatehealth.com/pdf/pomegranate/LE_Pomegranate_Reverses_Atherosclerosis_and_Slows_the_Progression_of_Prostate_Cancer.pdf

128. http://www.encognitive.com/files/Is%20Conventional%20Pomegranate%20Extract%20Enough_1.pdf

129. Kim, Dong-Heui, et al. "The Liver Protecting Effect of Pomegranate (Punica granatum) Seed Oil in Mice Treated with $ CCL_4$." *Applied Microscopy* 36.3 (2006): 173-182.

130. http://www.esnsa-eg.com/download/researchFiles/(11)%2053-2013.pdf

131. http://www.ijpcsonline.com/files/3-233.pdf

132. Fredericks, Charissa H., et al. "High-anthocyanin strawberries through cultivar selection." *Journal of the Science of Food and Agriculture* 93.4 (2013): 846-852.

133. Giampieri, Francesca, et al. "The strawberry: composition, nutritional quality, and impact on human health." *Nutrition* 28.1 (2012): 9-19.

134. Lau, Francis C., Barbara Shukitt-Hale, and James A. Joseph. "The beneficial effects of fruit polyphenols on brain aging." *Neurobiology of Aging* 26.1 (2005): 128-132.

135. http://journal.ashspublications.org/content/132/5/629.short

136. Mikulic-Petkovsek, Maja, et al. "Composition of sugars, organic acids, and total phenolics in 25 wild or cultivated berry species." *Journal of food science* 77.10 (2012): C1064-C1070.

137. Singh, Manjeet, et al. "Challenges for research on polyphenols from foods in Alzheimer's disease: bioavailability, metabolism, and cellular and molecular mechanisms." *Journal of agricultural and food chemistry* 56.13 (2008): 4855-4873.

138. Heo, Ho Jin, and Chang Yong Lee. "Strawberry and its anthocyanins reduce oxidative stress-induced apoptosis in PC12 cells." *Journal of agricultural and food chemistry* 53.6 (2005): 1984-1989.

139. Feng, Ying, et al. "Ellagic acid promotes Aβ42 fibrillization and inhibits Aβ42-induced neurotoxicity." *Biochemical and biophysical research communications* 390.4 (2009): 1250-1254.

140. Wang, Shiow Y., and Hsin-Shan Lin. "Antioxidant activity in fruits and leaves of blackberry, raspberry, and strawberry varies with cultivar and developmental stage." *Journal of agricultural and food chemistry* 48.2 (2000): 140-146.

141. Basu, Arpita, and Timothy J. Lyons. "Strawberries, blueberries, and cranberries in the metabolic syndrome: clinical perspectives." *Journal of agricultural and food chemistry* 60.23 (2011): 5687-5692.

142. Burton-Freeman, Britt, et al. "Strawberry modulates LDL oxidation and postprandial lipemia in response to high-fat meal in overweight hyperlipidemic men and women." *Journal of the American College of Nutrition* 29.1 (2010): 46-54.

143. Basu, Arpita, et al. "Strawberries decrease atherosclerotic markers in subjects with metabolic syndrome." *Nutrition research* 30.7 (2010): 462-469.

144. Naemura A, Mitani T, Ijiri Y, et al. Anti-thrombotic effect of strawberries. Blood Coagul Fibrinolysis. 2005 Oct;16(7):501-9.

145. http://www.actahort.org/books/626/626_2.htm

146. Shukitt-Hale B, Carey AN, Jenkins D, Rabin BM, Joseph JA. Beneficial effects of fruit extracts on neuronal function and behavior in a rodent model of accelerated aging. Neurobiol Aging. 2007 Aug;28(8):1187-94.

147. Törrönen, Riitta, et al. "Berries reduce postprandial insulin responses to wheat and rye breads in healthy women." *The Journal of nutrition* 143.4 (2013): 430-436.

148. Wang, Shiow Y., et al. "Resveratrol content in strawberry fruit is affected by preharvest conditions." *Journal of Agricultural and Food Chemistry* 55.20 (2007): 8269-8274.

149. https://www.cambridge.org/core/journals/british-journal-of-nutrition/article/postprandial-metabolic-events-and-fruit-derived-phenolics-a-review-of-the-science/EE10BBBA9C78CD-FACE16D1702916E9E7

150. http://biomedgerontology.oxfordjournals.org/content/early/2015/09/23/gerona.glv165.abstract

151. http://www.cranberryinstitute.org/HCP/05WinterNewsletter.pdf

152. Basu, Arpita, and Timothy J. Lyons. "Strawberries, blueberries, and cranberries in the metabolic syndrome: clinical perspectives." *Journal of agricultural and food chemistry* 60.23 (2011): 5687-5692.

153. http://link.springer.com/article/10.1007/s10096-007-0379-0

154. Jepson RG, Craig JC. A systematic review of the evidence for cranberries and blueberries in UTI prevention. MolNutr Food Res. 2007 Jun;51(6):738-45.

155. http://content.iospress.com/articles/biofactors/bio00819

156. Neto CC. Cranberry and its phytochemicals: a review of in vitro anticancer studies. J Nutr. 2007 Jan;137(1 Suppl):186S-93S

157. Lu KT, Chiou RY, Chen LG, et al. Neuroprotective effects of resveratrol on cerebral ischemia-induced neuron loss mediated by free radical scavenging and cerebral blood flow elevation. J Agric Food Chem. 2006 Apr 19;54(8):3126-31.

158. http://www.karger.com/Article/Fulltext/329181

159. Rimando, Agnes M., et al. "Resveratrol, pterostilbene, and piceatannol in vaccinium berries." *Journal of agricultural and food chemistry* 52.15 (2004): 4713-4719.

160. Joseph, James A., et al. "Cellular and behavioral effects of stilbene resveratrol analogues: implications for reducing the deleterious effects of aging." *Journal of agricultural and food chemistry* 56.22 (2008): 10544-10551.

161. http://www.lifeextension.com/magazine/2008/2/Maintaining-Youthful-Cognitive-Function-With-Blueberries/Page-01?p=1

162. http://pubs.acs.org/doi/abs/10.1021/jf203488k

163. http://www.lifeextension.com/magazine/2008/9/the-disease-fighting-power-of-berries/page-01?p=1

164. Seeram, Navindra P., et al. "Blackberry, black raspberry, blueberry, cranberry, red raspberry, and strawberry extracts inhibit growth and stimulate apoptosis of human cancer cells in vitro." *Journal of agricultural and food chemistry* 54.25 (2006): 9329-9339.

165. Häkkinen, S., et al. "Screening of selected flavonoids and phenolic acids in 19 berries." *Food Research International* 32.5 (1999): 345-353.

166. Wilms, Lonneke C., et al. "Protection by quercetin and quercetin-rich fruit juice against induction of oxidative DNA damage and formation of BPDE-DNA adducts in human lymphocytes." *Mutation Research/Genetic Toxicology and Environmental Mutagenesis* 582.1 (2005): 155-162.

167. Wang, Shiow Y., and Hsin-Shan Lin. "Antioxidant activity in fruits and leaves of blackberry, raspberry, and strawberry varies with cultivar and developmental stage." *Journal of agricultural and food chemistry* 48.2 (2000): 140-146.

168. http://pubs.acs.org/doi/abs/10.1021/jf9908345

169. Ross HA, McDougall GJ, Stewart D. Antiproliferative activity is predominantly associated with ellagitannins in raspberry extracts. Phytochemistry. 2007 Jan;68(2):218-28.

170. http://cancerpreventionresearch.aacrjournals.org/content/2/1/84.short

171. Ross, Heather A., Gordon J. McDougall, and Derek Stewart. "Antiproliferative activity is predominantly associated with ellagitannins in raspberry extracts." *Phytochemistry* 68.2 (2007): 218-228.

172. Mullen, William, et al. "Ellagitannins, flavonoids, and other phenolics in red raspberries and their contribution to antioxidant capacity and vasorelaxation properties." *Journal of Agricultural and Food Chemistry* 50.18 (2002): 5191-5196.

173. Mullen, William, et al. "Analysis of ellagitannins and conjugates of ellagic acid and quercetin in raspberry fruits by LC–MS n." *Phytochemistry* 64.2 (2003): 617-624.

174. Mullen, William, et al. "Effect of freezing and storage on the phenolics, ellagitannins, flavonoids, and antioxidant capacity of red raspberries." *Journal of Agricultural and Food Chemistry* 50.18 (2002): 5197-5201.

175. Borges, Gina, et al. "The bioavailability of raspberry anthocyanins and ellagitannins in rats." *Molecular nutrition & food research* 51.6 (2007): 714-725.

176. https://www.cambridge.org/core/journals/british-journal-of-nutrition/article/copper-and-iron-in-alzheimers-disease-a-systematic-review-and-its-dietary-implications/57BCD5F-F706594AD982363573AC75DFF

177. http://content.iospress.com/articles/journal-of-alzheimers-disease/jad140720

178. Ozarowski, Marcin, et al. "Rosmarinus officinalis L. leaf extract improves memory impairment and affects acetylcholinesterase and butyrylcholinesterase activities in rat brain." *Fitoterapia* 91 (2013): 261-271.

179. Al-Sereiti, M. R., K. M. Abu-Amer, and P. Sena. "Pharmacology of rosemary (Rosmarinus officinalis Linn.) and its therapeutic potentials." (1999).

180. Rasoolijazi, H., et al. "The protective role of carnosic acid against beta-amyloid toxicity in rats." *The Scientific World Journal* 2013 (2013).

181. Moreno, Silvia, et al. "Antioxidant and antimicrobial activities of rosemary extracts linked to their polyphenol composition." *Free radical research* 40.2 (2006): 223-231.

182. Hernández-Hernández, E., et al. "Antioxidant effect rosemary (Rosmarinus officinalis L.) and oregano (Origanum vulgare L.) extracts on TBARS and colour of model raw pork batters." *Meat Science* 81.2 (2009): 410-417.

183. Haraguchi, Hiroyuki, et al. "Inhibition of lipid peroxidation and superoxide generation by diterpenoids from Rosmarinus officinalis." *Planta Medica* 61.04 (1995): 333-336.

184. Moss, Mark, et al. "Aromas of rosemary and lavender essential oils differentially affect cognition and mood in healthy adults." *International Journal of Neuroscience* 113.1 (2003): 15-38.

185. Sasaki, Kazunori, et al. "Rosmarinus officinalis polyphenols produce anti-depressant like effect through monoaminergic and cholinergic functions modulation." *Behavioural brain research* 238 (2013): 86-94.

186. Park, Se-Eun, et al. "Neuroprotective effect of Rosmarinus officinalis extract on human dopaminergic cell line, SH-SY5Y." *Cellular and molecular neurobiology* 30.5 (2010): 759-767.

187. Machado, Daniele G., et al. "Rosmarinus officinalis L. hydroalcoholic extract, similar to fluoxetine, reverses depressive-like behavior without altering learning deficit in olfactory bulbectomized mice." *Journal of ethnopharmacology* 143.1 (2012): 158-169.

188. Bakırel, Tülay, et al. "In vivo assessment of antidiabetic and antioxidant activities of rosemary (Rosmarinus officinalis) in alloxan-diabetic rabbits." *Journal of ethnopharmacology* 116.1 (2008): 64-73.

189. Lucarini, Rodrigo, et al. "In vivo analgesic and anti-inflammatory activities of Rosmarinus officinalis aqueous extracts, rosmarinic acid and its acetyl ester derivative." *Pharmaceutical biology* 51.9 (2013): 1087-1090.

190. http://nutritionandmetabolism.biomedcentral.com/articles/10.1186/1743-7075-10-19

191. Al-Jamal, Abdul-Rahim, and Taha Alqadi. "Effects of rosemary (Rosmarinus officinalis) on lipid profile of diabetic rats." *Jordan Journal of Biological Sciences* 4.4 (2011): 199-204.

192. Ho, Chi-Tang, et al. "Chemistry and antioxidative factors in rosemary and sage." *Biofactors* 13.1-4 (2000): 161-166.

193. Bozin, Biljana, et al. "Antimicrobial and antioxidant properties of rosemary and sage (Rosmarinus officinalis L. and Salvia officinalis L., Lamiaceae) essential oils." *Journal of agricultural and food chemistry* 55.19 (2007): 7879-7885.

194. Abutbul, S., et al. "Use of Rosmarinus officinalis as a treatment against Streptococcus iniae in tilapia (Oreochromis sp.)." *Aquaculture* 238.1 (2004): 97-105.

195. Dastmalchi, Keyvan, et al. "Chemical composition and in vitro antioxidative activity of a lemon balm (Melissa officinalis L.) extract." *LWT-Food Science and Technology* 41.3 (2008): 391-400.and in vitro antioxidative activity of a lemon balm (Melissa officinalis L.) extract." *LWT-Food Science and Technology* 41.3 (2008): 391-400.

196. Lin, Jau-Tien, et al. "Antioxidant, anti-proliferative and cyclooxygenase-2 inhibitory activities of ethanolic extracts from lemon balm (Melissa officinalis L.) leaves." *LWT-Food Science and Technology* 49.1 (2012): 1-7.

197. Kennedy, D. O., et al. "Modulation of mood and cognitive performance following acute administration of Melissa officinalis (lemon balm)." *Pharmacology Biochemistry and Behavior* 72.4 (2002): 953-964.

198. Abuhamdah, Sawsan, and Paul L. Chazot. "Lemon Balm and Lavender herbal essential oils: Old and new ways to treat emotional disorders?." *Current Anaesthesia & Critical Care* 19.4 (2008): 221-226.

199. .http://journals.lww.com/psychosomaticmedicine/Abstract/2004/07000/Attenuation_of_Laboratory_Induced_Stress_in_Humans.22.aspx

200. http://www.wholehealthmedia.com/Melissa%20officinalis%20article.pdf

201. Guginski, Giselle, et al. "Mechanisms involved in the antinociception caused by ethanolic extract obtained from the leaves of Melissa officinalis (lemon balm) in mice." *Pharmacology Biochemistry and Behavior* 93.1 (2009): 10-16.

202. Perry, Elaine K., et al. "Medicinal plants and Alzheimer's disease: Integrating ethnobotanical and contemporary scientific evidence." *The Journal of Alternative and Complementary Medicine* 4.4 (1998): 419-428.

203. Houghton, P. J., and M-J. Howes. "Natural products and derivatives affecting neurotransmission relevant to Alzheimer's and Parkinson's disease." *Neurosignals* 14.1-2 (2005): 6-22.

204. http://ijp-online.com/article.asp?issn=0253-7613;year=2012;volume=44;issue=2;spage=189;epage=192;aulast=Taiwo

205. Yoo, Dae Young, et al. "Effects of Melissa officinalis L.(lemon balm) extract on neurogenesis associated with serum corticosterone and GABA in the mouse dentate gyrus." *Neurochemical research* 36.2 (2011): 250-257.

206. Miroliaei, Mehran, et al. "Inhibitory effects of Lemon balm (Melissa officinalis, L.) extract on the formation of advanced glycation end products." *Food Chemistry* 129.2 (2011): 267-271.

207. Kamdem, Jean Paul, et al. "Antioxidant activity, genotoxicity and cytotoxicity evaluation of lemon balm (Melissa officinalis L.) ethanolic extract: Its potential role in neuroprotection." *Industrial Crops and Products* 51 (2013): 26-34.

208. http://tih.sagepub.com/content/early/2010/09/20/0748233710383889.abstract

209. Mazzanti, G., et al. "Inhibitory activity of Melissa officinalis L. extract on Herpes simplex virus type 2 replication." *Natural product research* 22.16 (2008): 1433-1440.

210. http://www.taconicpharmacy.com/ns/DisplayMonograph.asp?storeID=78d7d29aa542412b949380f950889c3f&DocID=thyme

211. http://ijmr.org.in/article.asp?issn=0971-5916;year=2014;volume=139;issue=1;spage=1;epage=3;aulast=Pomponi

212. Youdim, Kuresh A., and Stanley G. Deans. "Beneficial effects of thyme oil on age-related changes in the phospholipid C 20 and C 22 polyunsaturated fatty acid composition of various rat tissues." *Biochimica et Biophysica Acta (BBA)-Molecular and Cell Biology of Lipids* 1438.1 (1999): 140-146.s

213. http://www.tandfonline.com/doi/abs/10.4081/ijas.2011.e20

214.
http://www.tandfonline.com/doi/abs/10.3109/09637486.2011.562882

215. Airoldi, Cristina, et al. "Natural compounds against Alzheimer's disease: molecular recognition of Aβ1–42 peptide by salvia sclareoides extract and its major component, rosmarinic acid, as investigated by NMR." *Chemistry–An Asian Journal* 8.3 (2013): 596-602.

216. http://onlinelibrary.wiley.com/doi/10.1002/cbf.3014/full

217. http://pubs.acs.org/doi/abs/10.1021/jf204902w

218. Pomponi, Massimiliano, and Massimo FL Pomponi. "Alzheimer's disease prevention & acetyl salicylic acid: a believable story." *Indian Journal of Medical Research* 139.1 (2014): 1.

219.
http://www.sciencedirect.com/science/article/pii/S0278691509002245

220. http://www.esnsa-eg.com/download/research-
Files/(5)%20%20%20%20115%20-%202015%20Assess-
ment%20of%20Radiation%20for%20brain%20.pdf

221. http://www.bioone.org/doi/abs/10.2987/8756-
971X(2005)21%5B80:MFTTVA%5D2.0.CO%3B2

222. Panickar, Kiran S., and Richard A. Anderson. "Effect of polyphenols on oxidative stress and mitochondrial dysfunction in neuronal death and brain edema in cerebral ischemia." *International journal of molecular sciences* 12.11 (2011): 8181-8207.

223. https://inis.iaea.org/search/search.aspx?orig_q=RN:44113179

224. http://het.sagepub.com/content/27/3/215.short

225. Aydın, Sevtap, A. Ahmet Başaran, and Nurşen Başaran. "Modulating effects of thyme and its major ingredients on oxidative DNA damage in human lymphocytes." *Journal of agricultural and food chemistry* 53.4 (2005): 1299-1305.

226. http://uokufa.edu.iq/journals/index.php/kjvs/article/view/2408

227. http://www.jsirjournal.com/Vol2Issue301.pdf

228. Charles, Denys J. "Thyme." *Antioxidant Properties of Spices, Herbs and Other Sources.* Springer New York, 2012. 553-561.

229. http://worldwidejournals.in/ojs/index.php/ijar/article/view/1673

230. Fuselli, Sandra R., et al. "Efficacy of indigenous plant essential oil Andean thyme (Acantholippia seriphioides A. Gray) to control American foulbrood (AFB) in honey bee (Apis mellifera L.) hives." *Journal of Essential Oil Research* 19.6 (2007): 514-519.

231. http://www.sciencedirect.com/science/
article/pii/S0308814609003124

232. http://www.mdpi.com/1420-3049/15/5/3200

233. Fecka, Izabela, and Sebastian Turek. "Determination of polyphenolic compounds in commercial herbal drugs and spices from Lamiaceae: thyme, wild thyme and sweet marjoram by chromatographic tech-niques." *Food Chemistry* 108.3 (2008): 1039-1053.

234. http://content.iospress.com/articles/journal-of-alzheimers-
disease/jad01083

235. http://www.alzheimers.net/2014-07-02/cinnamon-prevents-alzheimers/

236. George, Roshni C., John Lew, and Donald J. Graves. "Interaction of cinnamaldehyde and epicatechin with tau: implications of beneficial effects in modulating Alzheimer's disease pathogenesis." *Journal of Alzheimer's Disease* 36.1 (2013): 21-40.

237. http://journals.plos.org/plosone/article?id=10.1371/journal.pone.0016564

238. Couturier, Karine, et al. "Cinnamon intake alleviates the combined effects of dietary-induced insulin resistance and acute stress on brain mitochondria." *The Journal of nutritional biochemistry* 28 (2016): 183-190.

239. http://dst.sagepub.com/content/4/3/685.short

240. http://pubs.acs.org/doi/abs/10.1021/jf073065v

241. http://www.nature.com/aps/journal/vaop/ncurrent/full/aps201629a.html

242. Tabak, Mina, Robert Armon, and Ishak Neeman. "Cinnamon extracts' inhibitory effect on Helicobacter pylori." *Journal of ethnopharmacology* 67.3 (1999): 269-277.

243. Panickar, Kiran S., Marilyn M. Polansky, and Richard A. Anderson. "Cinnamon polyphenols attenuate cell swelling and mitochondrial dysfunction following oxygen-glucose deprivation in glial cells." *Experimental neurology* 216.2 (2009): 420-427.

244. http://www.fasebj.org/content/22/1_Supplement/700.8.short

245. Ho, Su-Chen, Ku-Shang Chang, and Pei-Wen Chang. "Inhibition of neuroinflammation by cinnamon and its main components." *Food chemistry* 138.4 (2013): 2275-2282.

246. http://bmccancer.biomedcentral.com/articles/10.1186/1471-2407-10-210

247. Pahan, Priyanka, and Kalipada Pahan. "Can cinnamon bring aroma in Parkinson's disease treatment?." *Neural regeneration research* 10.1 (2015): 30.

248. http://www.sciencedirect.com/science/article/pii/S2214750014000158

249.
http://www.sciencedirect.com/science/article/pii/S2214750014001073

250. http://www.fasebj.org/content/28/1_Supplement/830.11.short

251. Karuppagounder, Saravanan S., et al. "Dietary supplementation with resveratrol reduces plaque pathology in a transgenic model of Alzheimer's disease." *Neurochemistry international* 54.2 (2009): 111-118.

252. http://bmcneurosci.biomedcentral.com/articles/10.1186/1471-2202-9-S2-S6

253. http://www.jbc.org/content/280/45/37377.short

254. Anekonda, Thimmappa S. "Resveratrol—a boon for treating Alzheimer's disease?." *Brain research reviews* 52.2 (2006): 316-326.

255. http://onlinelibrary.wiley.com/doi/10.1111/j.1749-6632.2010.05865.x/full

256. Poulose, Shibu M., et al. "Effects of pterostilbene and resveratrol on brain and behavior." *Neurochemistry international* 89 (2015): 227-233.

257. https://www.jstage.jst.go.jp/article/bpb/37/6/37_b14-00022/_article

258. http://www.ingentaconnect.com/content/ben/cn-samc/2010/00000010/00000003/art00004

259. Vinutha, B., et al. "Screening of selected Indian medicinal plants for acetylcholinesterase inhibitory activity." *Journal of ethnopharmacology* 109.2 (2007): 359-363.

260. http://journals.lww.com/neuroreport/Abstract/2000/06260/Dendrite_extension_by_methanol_extract_of.35.aspx

261. https://www.degruyter.com/view/j/dmdi.2003.19.3/dmdi.2003.19.3.211/dmdi.2003.19.3.211.xml

262. Bhattacharya, A., S. Ghosal, and S. K. Bhattacharya. "Anti-oxidant effect of Withania somnifera glycowithanolides in chronic footshock stress-induced perturbations of oxidative free radical scavenging enzymes and lipid peroxidation in rat frontal cortex and striatum." *Journal of Ethnopharmacology* 74.1 (2001): 1-6.

263. http://www.sciencedirect.com/science/article/pii/S037887419800107X

264. Bhattacharya, S. K., and A. V. Muruganandam. "Adaptogenic activity of Withania somnifera: an experimental study using a rat model of chronic stress." *Pharmacology Biochemistry and Behavior* 75.3 (2003): 547-555.

265. Mirjalili, Mohammad Hossein, et al. "Steroidal lactones from Withania somnifera, an ancient plant for novel medicine." *Molecules* 14.7 (2009): 2373-2393.

266. http://journals.plos.org/plosone/article?id=10.1371/journal.pone.0077189

267. https://kevaind.org/download/Withania%20somnifera%20in%20Thyroid.pdf

268. http://www.pnas.org/content/109/9/3510.short

269. Kurapati, Kesava Rao Venkata, et al. "Ashwagandha (Withania somnifera) reverses β-amyloid 1-42 induced toxicity in human neuronal cells: implications in HIV-associated neurocognitive disorders (HAND)." *PLoS One* 8.10 (2013): e77624.

270. http://search.proquest.com/openview/91d8b2a4d7a4a60ae181fd269f6dfc72/1?pq-origsite=gscholar

271. Konar, Arpita, et al. "Protective role of Ashwagandha leaf extract and its component withanone on scopolamine-induced changes in the brain and brain-derived cells." *PloS one* 6.11 (2011): e27265.

272. http://journals.lww.com/neuroreport/Abstract/2002/10070/Axon__or_dendrite_predominant_outgrowth_induced_by.5.aspx

273. http://bmccomplementalternmed.biomedcentral.com/articles/10.1186/1472-6882-11-65

274. http://www.ajol.info/index.php/ajtcam/article/view/67963

275. http://journals.lww.com/neuroreport/Abstract/2002/10070/Axon__or_dendrite_predominant_outgrowth_induced_by.5.aspx

276. Joseph, James A., Barbara Shukitt-Hale, and Lauren M. Willis. "Grape juice, berries, and walnuts affect brain aging and behavior." *The Journal of nutrition* 139.9 (2009): 1813S-1817S.

277. http://www.jneurosci.org/content/29/41/12795.short

278. Essa, Musthafa M., et al. "Neuroprotective effect of natural products against Alzheimer's disease." *Neurochemical research* 37.9 (2012): 1829-1842.

279. Poulose, Shibu M., Donna F. Bielinski, and Barbara Shukitt-Hale. "Walnut diet reduces accumulation of polyubiquitinated proteins and inflammation in the brain of aged rats." *The Journal of nutritional biochemistry* 24.5 (2013): 912-919.

280. Muthaiyah, Balu, et al. "Protective effects of walnut extract against amyloid beta peptide-induced cell death and oxidative stress in PC12 cells." *Neurochemical research* 36.11 (2011): 2096-2103.

281. http://content.iospress.com/articles/journal-of-alzheimers-disease/jad140675

282. http://www.ingentaconnect.com/content/ben/car/2004/00000001/00000003/art00006

283. https://www.ncbi.nlm.nih.gov/books/NBK11893/?report=reader

284. Bourre, Jean-Marie. "Omega-3 fatty acids in psychiatry." *Medecine sciences: M/S* 21.2 (2005): 216-221.

285. http://www.ingentaconnect.com/content/ben/car/2013/00000010/00000006/art00009

286. Carey, Amanda N., et al. "The ability of walnut extract and fatty acids to protect against the deleterious effects of oxidative stress and inflammation in hippocampal cells." *Nutritional neuroscience* 16.1 (2013): 13-20.

287. http://www.tandfonline.com/doi/abs/10.3109/09637486.2011.585964